The British Medical Association
FAMILY DOCTOR GUIDE *to*
CANCER

D0294024

The British Medical Association

FAMILY DOCTOR GUIDE *to*

CANCER

DR. GARETH REES

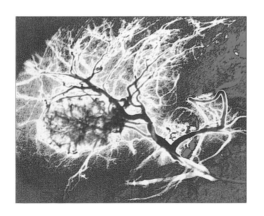

MEDICAL EDITOR
DR. TONY SMITH

A DORLING KINDERSLEY BOOK

IMPORTANT

This book is intended not as a substitute for personal medical advice but as a supplement to that advice for the patient who wishes to understand more about his/her condition.

Before taking any form of treatment YOU SHOULD ALWAYS CONSULT YOUR MEDICAL PRACTITIONER.

In particular (without limit) you should note that advances in medical science occur rapidly and some of the information about drugs and treatment contained in this book may very soon be out of date.

PLEASE NOTE
The author regrets that she cannot enter into any correspondence with readers.

DORLING KINDERSLEY
LONDON, NEW YORK, SYDNEY, DELHI, PARIS,
MUNICH AND JOHANNESBURG

DK www.dk.com

Senior Editor Mary Lindsay
Senior Art Editor Janice English
Production Controller Heather Hughes
Managing Editor Martyn Page
Managing Art Editor Bryn Walls

Produced for Dorling Kindersley Limited by
Design Revolution, Queens Park Villa,
30 West Drive, Brighton, East Sussex BN2 2GE
Editorial Director Ian Whitelaw
Art Director Becky Willis
Editor Julie Whitaker
Designer Fiona Roberts

Published in Great Britain in 2000 by
Dorling Kindersley Limited,
9 Henrietta Street, London WC2E 8PS

2 4 6 8 10 9 7 5 3 1

A CIP catalogue record for this book is available from the British Library

ISBN 0-7513-0816-1

Reproduced by Colourscan, Singapore
Printed in Hong Kong by Wing King Tong

Contents

Dedicated to
my parents

Introduction

*O*ne in three of us will develop cancer. There are now roughly two million people in Britain who have had treatment for cancer, more than one in 25 of the population. The majority of these are long-term survivors. Attitudes are changing, and for most people cancer is no longer the taboo subject that it used to be. Many people who have cancer now find it easier to talk about their diagnosis, in the same way they would about most other illnesses.

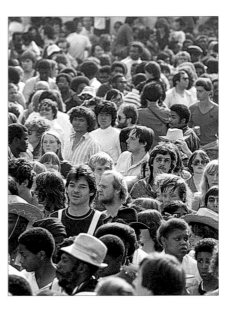

You may already be aware that advances in medical science have had a major impact on the outlook for people with cancer. Of course the news is not all good, but as we enter the new millennium, the future for many cancer patients is now rather more hopeful than for many of those with other illnesses that traditionally have been much less feared. We are rapidly learning more about what exactly goes wrong when cells become cancerous, and these discoveries will lead to more exciting new treatments in the fairly near future.

Cancer became increasingly common during the 20th century. One reason is that there are more of us in the

A COMMON DISEASE
Approximately one in three people who live in the UK will develop cancer during their lifetime.

older age range and cancer tends to be a disease of older people. The other main cause has been smoking. However, although cancer has become more common, at the same time the chances of a cure have also steadily increased. Even those people whose cancer cannot yet be cured are living longer and have a better quality of life.

Improvements have occurred as a result of earlier diagnosis, better treatments, better supportive care and better organisation. Anyone who has cancer should now expect to receive 'state of the art' treatment as well as having access to wide-ranging support from both the NHS and many charitable and voluntary organisations.

This book does not deal with the causes of cancer nor does it discuss particular cancers in detail, but it aims to give a brief introduction to what is known about the nature of cancer, what can now be done for people who get it, and what treatment and care in general are likely to involve. It is worth mentioning that the study of everything to do with cancer is known as oncology – *onkos* is the Greek word for lump.

This book has been written for anyone who has cancer and their families and friends, in the hope that they will find it informative, helpful and easy to understand.

KEY POINTS

- Cancer is common: one in three people can expect to develop some form of the disease.
- Treatment for cancer is improving all the time.

What is cancer?

Cancer is not a single illness: there are very many different types. Some cancers may stay almost unchanged for several years and have no impact on life expectancy. By contrast, there are rare cancers that may prove fatal shortly after they have been discovered. In the same way that the term 'infection' embraces illnesses as far apart as the common cold, a boil, malaria and tuberculosis, the spectrum of malignant disease is almost equally varied, in both behaviour and seriousness.

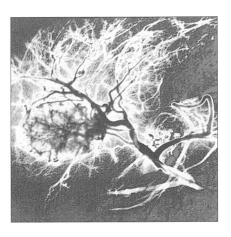

LIVER TUMOUR
This contrast X-ray shows the blood vessels in a liver tumour. Tumour cells have stimulated the growth of new blood vessels, which 'feed' the tumour, encouraging further enlargement. Much current research is aimed towards developing new treatments designed to block this process.

LOSS OF CONTROL

A lump of human tissue the size of a sugar cube may contain a thousand million cells. These are the minute building blocks from which our bodies are made, visible only down the microscope. It is quite amazing that the billions of cells in a human body normally function in perfect harmony, every cell knowing its place and doing the job that it was designed to do. Most cells have a finite lifespan: millions of new ones are produced every day to replace those lost through old age or wear and tear.

New cells are produced when existing cells divide into two, a process known as 'mitosis'. Except in children, who are growing, there is normally a perfect balance between the numbers of the cells that are dying and those that are dividing. Normally exactly the right amounts of new cells are produced to replace those that are being lost. The control mechanisms involved are very complex. Loss of control can lead to an excess of cells, resulting in a tumour.

However, it is important to realise that only a small minority of tumours are cancerous. Most tumours are localised accumulations of normal or fairly normal cells and are benign. A wart is a common example.

The development of a cancer involves a change in the quality of the cells as well as an increase in quantity: they change in both appearance and behaviour. They become more aggressive, destructive and independent of normal cells. They acquire the ability to infiltrate and invade the surrounding tissues. In some instances, the cells may also invade lymphatic and blood vessels and thus spread away from the 'primary' growth to other places. In time, these cells may cause the development of secondary growths, known as 'metastases', in the lymph glands and other organs such as lungs, liver and bones.

GENES

The behaviour of all cells is controlled by genes in their central control unit, the nucleus. Each cell nucleus contains approximately 100,000 genes. The genes are minute highly concentrated packets of information and instructions stored in coded form in a complex chemical molecule known as 'DNA'. Large numbers of genes are grouped together in strands looking rather like short pieces of string, which are just visible under the microscope. These are the chromosomes, which are joined to each other in pairs, 23 pairs in total.

Genetic Material

All cells in the body (except for sperm and eggs) have a full complement of genetic material in the form of 23 pairs of chromosomes. Each chromosome is a coiled double strand of helical DNA that makes up a sequence of genes

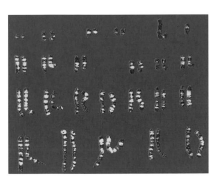

CHROMOSOMES IN A
SINGLE HUMAN CELL

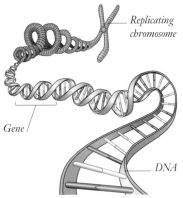

Replicating chromosome

Gene

DNA

UNRAVELLED CHROMOSOME

A human being develops in the uterus from a single cell. This first cell is formed by the fertilisation of an ovum (egg) produced in one of the mother's ovaries by a sperm produced in one of the father's testes. It divides to produce two 'daughter' cells and then these both divide, resulting in four cells. Successive divisions lead to rapid growth. Mitosis involves replication of all the genetic information so that every one of the cells in the developing microscopic organism or 'embryo' has its own full complement. This process of replication and division continues as the embryo develops into a 'fetus' and then eventually into a newborn baby.

The genetic information contained within the first cell is what determines the physical characteristics of the whole human being that ultimately develops from it.

However, once the body is fully formed, most of this genetic information is no longer required by any particular individual cell. All it needs is the information required to enable it to perform its own designated role. Instructions on how to perform other roles are redundant. The important pieces of information that are 'switched on' in particular cells govern the characteristics and behaviour of those cells and the properties of the particular tissues that they constitute.

CANCER GENES

There are particular genes known as 'oncogenes', which are present in normal cells where they may either be dormant or play a part in controlling cell behaviour and division.

Genetic Damage

Oncogenes and tumour suppressor genes regulate cell division. Damage to these genes by carcinogens is usually repaired, but accumulated unrepaired damage to several genes can cause the cell to lose its normal function and become cancerous.

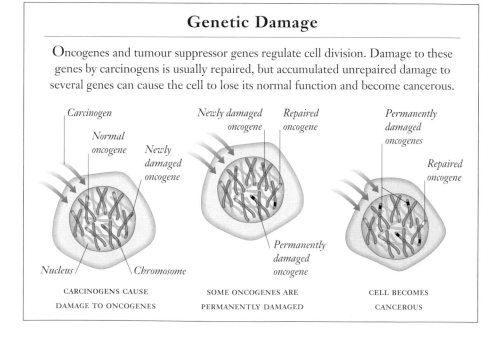

CARCINOGENS CAUSE
DAMAGE TO ONCOGENES

SOME ONCOGENES ARE
PERMANENTLY DAMAGED

CELL BECOMES
CANCEROUS

DNA damage caused, for example, by tobacco smoke, ultraviolet light or certain viruses can trigger certain abnormalities or 'mutations' in these genes, resulting in increased and abnormal activity of the gene. This can cause the cell to behave in an antisocial way and to become malignant (i.e. cancerous).

In addition to oncogenes, each cell contains 'tumour suppressor genes' whose normal job is to restrain it from dividing. Many cancers are caused by damage that reduces the activity of a tumour suppressor gene.

Genes are crucial not only to the development of malignancy, but also to the subsequent behaviour of a cancer and its response to treatment. For example, some genes are responsible for the manufacture of proteins important for a cancer's ability to invade adjacent tissues and to spread to distant parts of the body, triggering the development of metastases. Other genes can cause the cell to produce self-stimulating 'growth factors' or to eliminate anti-cancer drugs.

Even the process of cell death is under genetic control. Genetic damage may result in cells failing to die, which can be an important factor both in the development of a cancer and in its resistance to treatment with radiotherapy or drugs.

The development of a cancer involves an accumulation of successive genetic abnormalities over some years, both before and after the cells start behaving in a malignant fashion. Further gene mutations after the cancer has started can result in some of the cancerous cells behaving differently from others. This may cause the growth to 'change its spots' at some stage.

The behaviour of the cancer and the long-term result of treatment depend ultimately on those cells that have

How a Tumour Forms

A cancerous tumour begins as a single cell. If it is not destroyed by the body's immune system, it will divide into two cells, which in turn divide into four and so on. After only four cell divisions, a cancerous growth will contain 16 cells.

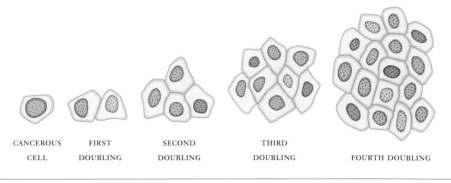

| CANCEROUS CELL | FIRST DOUBLING | SECOND DOUBLING | THIRD DOUBLING | FOURTH DOUBLING |

the most antisocial characteristics and on those that are best able to resist treatment aimed at destroying them.

SPEED OF GROWTH

Most cells divide at the most every few days, some much more slowly. Given that almost all cancers start off as a result of a genetic abnormality in a single cell, and that there may be a thousand million cells in a sugar cube-sized lump, it follows that most cancers begin a very long time before they become apparent. Most cancers are rather larger than the size of a sugar lump when they are discovered and many will by then have been present, growing slowly, for 10–20 years. There is, however, a large variation in the time a tumour takes to double in size. This 'doubling time' may vary from a few days to many years, although for most of the more common cancers the average is about 2–3 months.

EFFECTS OF CANCER

It can sometimes be difficult to understand just how an excessive number of abnormal cells can in certain circumstances be a threat to life. The serious effects of malignant disease occur as a result of progressive infiltration and destruction of the surrounding normal tissues and/or other parts of the body to which the cancer has spread, such as the liver, bones or lungs. It is unusual for localised cancers to be fatal. Most of those who die from cancer have widespread or metastatic disease. However, in addition to these 'physical' processes, cancers can cause progressive debilitation by producing a wide range of toxic chemicals acting both locally and, via the bloodstream, throughout the body. We do not understand this process fully, but it is these chemicals that can be responsible for symptoms such as loss of weight in some patients.

CLASSIFICATION OF CANCERS

Cancers are graded according to the extent to which the cells are different from normal. In well-differentiated (sometimes called 'grade 1') cancers some of the normal cellular architecture is maintained and the cells do not seem to be dividing frequently. Some may still be retaining some ability to perform their original specific tasks. At the other end of the spectrum are poorly differentiated ('grade 3') cancers in which the cells have changed so much that they are now very different from normal cells and have completely lost their ability to perform their appointed tasks. These cancers tend to be faster growing and more aggressive, and to carry a less favourable prognosis. Moderately differentiated cancers are in between.

Cancers are classified according to the type of normal cell from which they originated, not according to the tissues into which they may have spread. This is what might be called the primary classification. Cancers in each category will be graded as described above, and their growth and extent of spread will also be assessed in a process known as 'staging' (see pp.35–36).

As far as the primary classification of cancers is concerned, almost all cancers can be placed in one of the following groups.

CARCINOMAS

Carcinomas are by far the most common types of cancer. They originate from cells lining body surfaces, including the skin and a wide variety of internal linings. Among these are those of the mouth, throat, bronchi (the tubes carrying air in and out of the lungs), oesophagus (the swallowing tube or gullet), stomach, bowel, bladder, uterus (womb) and ovaries, and the linings of ducts in the breasts, prostate gland and pancreas.

There are different types of carcinomas named according to the appearance of the normal cells from which they arose. 'Squamous carcinomas' arise particularly in the skin, mouth, throat, oesophagus and lung; 'adenocarcinomas' arise particularly in the lower oesophagus, stomach, bowel, breast and ovary; 'transitional cell carcinomas' arise chiefly in the bladder and 'small cell carcinomas' also occur in the lung.

SARCOMAS

These arise from supportive rather than surface lining tissues, such as bone, fat, muscle and the strengthening 'fibrous tissue' found in most parts of the body.

LYMPHOMAS

These originate from cells known as 'lymphocytes', which are found throughout the body, particularly in the lymph glands and blood. Lymphocytes are a very important component of the body's immune system. Lymphomas are divided into 'Hodgkin's disease' and the 'non-Hodgkin's lymphomas', according to the cell type affected.

LEUKAEMIAS

Leukaemias arise from the cells in the bone marrow that make the white blood cells. The white blood cells are crucial to the body's defence system against infection. In leukaemia, there is a greatly increased concentration of abnormal white cells in the blood, which causes problems both because the abnormal cells often do not function properly and because they restrict the space within the bone marrow for new normal blood cells to be made.

MYELOMAS

These are malignancies of the 'plasma cells' in the bone marrow that produce antibodies – the proteins that help to fight infections.

GERM CELL TUMOURS

These develop from those cells in the testes and ovaries responsible for the production of ova and sperm. They include 'teratomas' and 'seminomas'.

MELANOMAS

These skin cancers arise from the skin pigment-producing cells or 'melanocytes'.

GLIOMAS

These develop from cells of the supporting tissue of the brain or spinal cord. They seldom metastasise.

PRE-CANCERS

It is important to mention the fairly common potentially pre-cancerous conditions, which are diagnosed mainly in apparently healthy people who undergo 'screening' tests such as cervical smears and mammograms (breast X-rays). These conditions particularly affect the surfaces of the cervix (neck of the womb) and breast ducts and are referred to as 'carcinoma in situ'.

This means that the cells on the very surface have a malignant appearance when seen though a microscope, but they show no sign of having begun to behave malignantly by invading any of the tissue immediately beneath the surface lining. Carcinoma in situ has no ability to spread via the lymphatic or blood systems and in itself poses absolutely no threat to life. It does, however, carry a risk of eventually becoming truly cancerous if left untreated.

KEY POINTS

- Cancers start off as a consequence of gene damage in a single cell and usually take many years to become apparent.
- Cancers vary enormously in appearance, behaviour and prognosis.

How is cancer diagnosed?

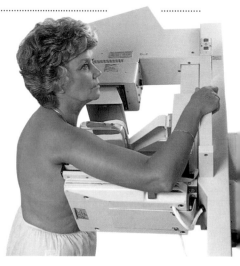

The great majority of cancers are discovered because of the symptoms that they cause, or because the person concerned (or their doctor) notices a lump or other abnormal appearance. A small but growing proportion of cancers are discovered as a result of doing tests on apparently healthy people who have noticed nothing abnormal. This is called 'screening'.

SCREENING FOR CANCER
All women over 50 are offered mammography every three years until they reach 65, and beyond on demand.

SYMPTOMS OF CANCER

Most of the symptoms that can be caused by cancer are far more commonly the result of relatively minor illnesses that have nothing to do with cancer. Sometimes this means that the individual concerned does not take them seriously to start with, and so delays seeking medical advice. Even when he or she does go to the doctor, the general practitioner may not always feel that it is appropriate to consider cancer very seriously as a possible diagnosis at this stage. There is really no way around this. Very thorough and immediate investigation of any symptom that might possibly be caused by a cancer would rapidly cause the health service to grind to a halt, not to mention causing a lot of unnecessary anxiety.

Your doctor is more likely to suspect the possibility of a potentially serious cause for a symptom if it persists, or if you have certain other symptoms as well. Some symptoms are sufficiently likely to have a serious explanation that they require further investigation as a routine matter.

LUMPS AND BUMPS

The majority of cancers are fairly deep-seated within the body and only a minority can be felt on examination by a

Suspicious Symptoms

Anyone who has any of the symptoms listed in the box should seek medical advice promptly. The majority of people with these symptoms will not have cancer, but it should be ruled out.

PERSISTENT AND UNEXPLAINED	ABNORMAL BLEEDING
Cough	Coughing up blood
Breathlessness	Rectal bleeding
Hoarse voice	Vaginal bleeding between periods
Difficulty with swallowing	
Pain	Vaginal bleeding with intercourse
Indigestion	
Weight loss	Postmenopausal vaginal bleeding
Altered bowel habit	
Discharge from any orifice (for example, nipple or vagina)	Blood in the urine
	Bleeding from a mole
Fever	

doctor, let alone by the patient. However, cancers that are nearer to the surface, such as those involving the breast or lymph glands in the neck or armpits, are often discovered by the person concerned becoming aware of a lump. Most skin cancers are also noticed first by the person concerned rather than by their doctor.

In fact, few lumps or persistent skin changes turn out to be cancerous. However, if you do notice a lump in the breast, testis or elsewhere, or if you have a persistent or worsening unexplained ulcer or 'spot', particularly any change in appearance of a mole, you should seek medical advice promptly.

SCREENING FOR CANCER

Screening to discover cancers at an early and more curable stage can help to reduce the number of deaths from a few important types of cancer. However, screening has its problems. If your test result shows up an abnormality that eventually turns out not to be cancer, as often happens, you will have had to go through further investigations and you may have experienced a lot of unnecessary worry.

Screening can sometimes reveal the presence of a slow-growing cancer or a pre-cancerous growth that would not in fact have caused any serious problems had it not been discovered. As a result some people may receive treatment that is not really necessary. Screening is expensive: usually a very large number of people have to be screened to discover one cancer for which earlier diagnosis makes the difference between the success and failure of treatment.

BREAST CANCER SCREENING

Women over the age of 50 are offered mammography (see p.33) every three years until they reach the age of 65,

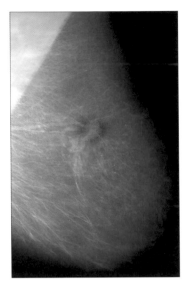

Breast Cancer
This coloured mammogram image of the breast shows a cancer (seen as a pink area). Mammographic screening can help detect cancers at an early stage, improving the chances of a cure.

and beyond on demand. The majority of abnormalities seen on the X-ray pictures are not cancerous, but further investigation of some of them is recommended, sometimes leading to the removal of a small piece of tissue (a 'biopsy') for microscopic analysis. A few of these abnormalities are then discovered to be cancerous or pre-cancerous. The breast cancers discovered in this way are usually small and mammographic screening has been shown to improve significantly the chance of cure.

Cervical Cancer Screening

Sexually active women should have a cervical smear test every 3–5 years up to the age of 60 to 65. (Women who have never had sexual intercourse very rarely get this type of cancer.) When you have a smear test an instrument called a speculum is inserted into the vagina to enable the cervix (neck of the womb) to be seen. The cervix is then scraped gently with a wooden spatula to collect a reasonable number of cells. These are smeared on to a piece of glass and examined under the microscope. The procedure may be a little uncomfortable, but is not normally painful. The test can discover pre-cancerous abnormalities that can be dealt with easily. It can also discover cancers at a very early stage, when treatment gives a high probability of cure.

Most of the abnormalities discovered in this way are only minor changes, which may require no further investigation, or merely a repeat smear or more frequent smears for a while. However, some abnormalities require further investigation in a procedure called 'colposcopy', which involves examining the illuminated cervix with a type of magnifying glass. Tiny samples or 'punch biopsies' can be removed from any abnormal areas. This is briefly uncomfortable, but it should not be painful and only lasts about 10 minutes.

If potentially pre-cancerous areas are discovered, further treatment to destroy the pre-cancerous cells is recommended. This may involve 'laser evaporation' (a concentrated beam of light vaporises the abnormal cells), 'cryotherapy' (the abnormal cells are destroyed with a freezing probe) under local anaesthetic or 'diathermy' (the abnormal cells are burnt by an electrical probe) under general anaesthetic.

In a small percentage of women, the colposcopy may suggest that the abnormality is more serious and a 'cone biopsy' (removal of the central lining of the cervical canal) under a general anaesthetic may be necessary. This may well remove all the affected tissue but, occasionally, a more deeply infiltrating growth is discovered that requires more extensive treatment.

Very few women die from cancer of the cervix and, of those who do, almost 90 per cent have never had a routine smear.

SCREENING FOR OTHER CANCERS

Recent research has shown that screening that detects bowel tumours at an early stage can cut the number of deaths from bowel cancer. This involves testing stool specimens for small amounts of blood that are not normally visible to the naked eye. Although the cause of such bleeding is usually something other than cancer, sometimes further investigation by colonoscopy or barium enema (see pp.32 and 33) will reveal the presence of a cancer before it has grown sufficiently to

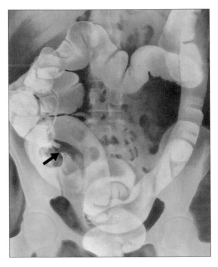

BARIUM ENEMA
This coloured contrast X-ray shows the bowel outlined by barium introduced as an enema. The arrow shows the location of a tumour.

cause symptoms. It seems likely that 'faecal occult blood' testing will become more widely available.

Screening for prostate cancer can be done by testing the blood for a chemical often produced by these cancers ('prostate-specific antigen' or 'PSA'), and by a physical examination and ultrasound scanning. Screening can detect some prostate cancers at an early stage, but it can also result in unnecessary treatment. The prostates of most old men dying from other conditions can be found to contain small cancers. Most cancers occurring in elderly people are slow growing and, if left untreated, are unlikely to cause problems during the remainder of an individual's life. However, recent evidence suggests that screening can reduce deaths from prostate cancer.

Screening for lung cancer by routine chest X-rays has not proved worthwhile. Most lung cancers appear to carry an unfavourable prognosis from an early stage and at present the best hope of reducing significantly deaths from this disease is through a reduction in smoking.

CANCER IN FAMILIES

In theory, it makes sense to screen people who are known (or who are likely) to have inherited a genetic predisposition to cancer. However, fewer than five per cent of cancers have an inherited cause. Cancer is a common disease and, when it affects two or more members of the same family, the strong probability is that this is pure chance. Occasionally it may be the result of a shared environmental factor such as smoking.

Hereditary cancer may be suspected when two or more close relatives – parents, brothers or sisters – have either the same cancer or different ones that can sometimes be genetically related, such as those of the breast and ovary. Other hallmarks are the development of the cancer at a young age and a tendency to have bilateral (in both breasts, for example) or multiple tumours.

Some of those with a strong family history may have inherited certain identifiable abnormal genes. If they have, it is, however, by no means certain that they will develop a cancer, although inheriting some genes can give an 80 to 90 per cent or even higher risk of developing cancer at some stage. The same type of cancer can sometimes occur in two or more members of a family without any particular genetic abnormality being identifiable. The risk for other members of the family may then be increased, but not usually to a high level.

A predisposition to a variety of rare cancers can be inherited, for example, certain tumours of the thyroid and other hormone-producing glands. As far as the more common types of cancer are concerned, the main types that are occasionally inherited are those of the large bowel (colon and rectum), the breast and the ovary.

Bowel cancer can occasionally run in families through inheritance of a mutated 'adenomatosis polyposis coli' (APC) gene. Affected individuals develop multiple benign bowel polyps at an early age and these subsequently become malignant in almost all cases.

Breast cancer is inherited in only 5–10 per cent of cases. So far two important breast cancer genes have been discovered: 'BRCA-1' and 'BRCA-2'. A woman who has inherited a mutated BRCA-1 or BRCA-2 gene has about an 85 per cent chance of developing breast cancer at some stage. The mutated BRCA-1 gene also confers an increased risk of ovarian cancer. However, most women with a family history of breast cancer do not have an inherited BRCA-1 or BRCA-2 mutation. They may be at an increased risk of breast cancer, but the level of risk is usually much lower, for example below 30 per cent for those with a mother or sister with the disease.

If you are worried that you may be at an increased risk of cancer because of your family history, you should discuss this with your own doctor. If appropriate you may be referred for a specialised opinion from a clinical geneticist who may well be able to reassure you that you are not at a significantly increased risk. Alternatively, it may be possible to arrive at an approximate assessment of the level of any increased risk.

Occasionally it is appropriate to test for the presence of an abnormal gene by very sophisticated analysis of a blood sample. However, this test is only performed if the individual concerned still wants it done after very detailed discussion of all the implications, which can be profound. These include consideration of what will be done if a cancer-predisposing gene is discovered, feelings about living with the certain knowledge of high risk of developing cancer, what other family members will be told, the consequences for parenthood and how eligibility for life insurance may be affected.

Recommendations as to what should be done for those individuals identified as being at high risk vary enormously according to the cancer concerned, individual circumstances and preferences. Someone who is facing a high risk of developing hereditary bowel cancer may well be advised to have their colon and rectum removed surgically in their teens or 20s, before the disease has had a chance to develop. When this is done, the small bowel can be joined to the anus, avoiding the need for a 'stoma' (see p.53).

For women with a high risk of breast cancer, choosing the best form of preventive treatment is less straight-forward. Some women will opt for prophylactic (that is, preventive) removal of both breasts (a bilateral mastectomy). However, although this procedure does seem to reduce significantly the chance of a woman developing breast cancer, there is no guarantee. A few women have developed cancer in the small amount of breast tissue that is left behind after mastectomy. Some women opt instead for a programme of close surveillance involving regular physical examination by a specialist and mammography.

Women who are at increased risk of ovarian cancer may opt to have both ovaries removed surgically as a preventive measure (bilateral 'oophorectomy'). However, this also is not guaranteed to prevent the disease. Screening to detect ovarian cancer at an early stage using ultrasound scanning and blood testing for the CA-125 'tumour marker' produced by this cancer is an alternative.

MEDICAL ASSESSMENT

If your symptoms suggest the possibility of cancer, or if your doctor finds something unusual during an examination or as the result of a screening test, you will probably need further assessment and tests, depending on the circumstances. Some further investigation may be arranged by your GP, but at some stage you are likely to be referred to a hospital consultant for an opinion on what should be done next. What is appropriate can vary greatly from one individual to another.

Waiting for appointments, further investigations and their results can inevitably be very worrying, but support is usually available from a variety of people and organisations (see Further Care, p.85, and Useful Addresses, p.116).

CLINICAL ASSESSMENT

If you do need further assessment, the first step is likely to be a consultation with a specialist in an outpatient clinic where you will be asked more detailed questions about any symptoms you may have, such as their severity and duration. You can also expect to be asked about your general health and other aspects that may be relevant, such as previous illnesses, any medication you may be taking, present or past occupations and your home circumstances. This 'history taking' will then usually be followed by a physical examination, which will tend to concentrate on the part of your body that is giving cause for concern, although you may also have a more generalised examination.

PHYSICAL EXAMINATION
Your doctor may find something suspicious during a physical examination that he/she feels needs further investigation.

This assessment does not always help in making a diagnosis, but sometimes the doctor will suspect that there is a cancer because he or she finds, for example, a lump that has particular suggestive features.

The examination that is carried out may include taking a look inside some part of your body. A variety of instruments may be used to examine, for example, the rectum (proctoscope), the voicebox (small mirrors), or the cervix (by inserting a speculum into the vagina).

FURTHER INVESTIGATIONS

If there is a suspicion of serious disease, further tests will probably be arranged. These may include biopsy, blood tests, X-rays and scans.

BIOPSY

Although a lump may feel or appear cancerous, a definite diagnosis of cancer can usually be made only by a pathologist, a doctor who specialises in assessing cells and tissues by studying them through a microscope. He or she will recognise the characteristic changes in appearance that confirm that cancer is present.

The removal of a piece of tissue for diagnostic purposes is known as a 'biopsy'. Part of a lump or, if feasible, a whole lump (excision biopsy) may be removed during an operation performed under local or general anaesthetic. Sometimes a thin core of tissue may be removed by a special type of needle device, which avoids the need to cut into tissue with a scalpel.

Alternatively, cells from the abnormal tissue may be sucked ('aspirated') into a thin needle attached to a syringe. This is called a 'fine needle aspiration biopsy' and, in most cases, is uncomfortable only very briefly. The cells can then be smeared on to a glass slide. Cells for microscopic examination can also be obtained by scraping the tissue concerned, as in cervical smear testing, or from tissue fluids such as sputum, fluid surrounding the lung ('pleural effusion') or urine.

The microscopic examination of very thin processed slices taken from a lump of tissue is known as 'histology', whereas the examination of a cellular smear is known as 'cytology'. Histology can provide more detailed information because the pathologist is able to assess not

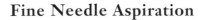

Fine Needle Aspiration

Cells are withdrawn from the area of the lump using a syringe with a fine needle. This diagram shows a needle aspiration of the thyroid gland. The micrograph image shows cancerous thyroid cells that have been removed by this procedure.

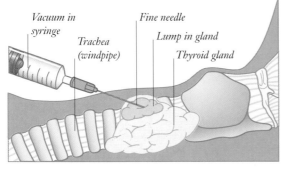

Vacuum in syringe

Trachea (windpipe)

Fine needle

Lump in gland

Thyroid gland

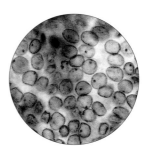

TAKING A SAMPLE

CANCEROUS THYROID CELLS

only the appearance of individual cells (that is to say, the bricks) but also the relationships between cells and the way in which the tissue is constructed (the architecture).

Cytology is based on the appearance of individual cells. It is capable of establishing the presence of a cancerous process but gives less qualitative information than histology. It also suffers from the potential problem that the cells removed from abnormal tissue by fine needle aspiration may not be representative – the needle may not have sucked up any cancerous cells, even though some were actually present. This risk of a 'false-negative' result is not usually a problem with histology. However, a positive cytology result is usually sufficient to justify setting in train further treatment. For many cancers, this treatment will involve surgical removal, when tissue will become available for histological examination.

In addition to microscopic examination of tissue to establish the diagnosis, biopsies are also sometimes performed in an attempt to establish the extent of the disease. For example, someone who has a swollen neck gland diagnosed as lymphoma may undergo a bone marrow biopsy to see whether there are lymphoma cells in the marrow, because this could influence significantly the choice of treatment.

DIAGNOSTIC INSTRUMENTS

The term '-oscopy' merely means 'taking a look' (*skopein* is Greek for 'to see'). Most cancers arise from the inner lining of tubes or containers such as the voice box (the larynx), air passages in the lungs (the bronchi), swallowing tube or gullet (the oesophagus), stomach (for which the medical adjective is 'gastric'), large bowel (the colon and rectum) and bladder (sometimes referred to as 'cyst'). It is possible to inspect all of these structures using a variety of instruments and to take biopsies from any suspicious areas.

Many inspections now involve the use of fibreoptic technology, which enables the doctor to see down a flexible cable inserted gently into the relevant opening in the body, or through a small cut. Sometimes it is easier for your doctor to see, feel and assess the extent of the growth, and to take a biopsy while you are under a general anaesthetic. This is why examination under anaesthetic (EUA) is quite a common procedure.

BLOOD TESTS

These are unlikely to provide the doctor with much useful information to help make the diagnosis unless the malignancy is of the white blood cells themselves

Types of Investigation

The names and the organs involved in some investigations are listed below. Some investigations take place in the outpatient clinic, while others require sedation or a general anaesthetic.

Laryngoscopy	Voice box
Bronchoscopy	Lungs
Gastroscopy	Stomach
Colonoscopy	Colon
Sigmoidoscopy	The S-shaped lower end of the colon and rectum
Cystoscopy	Bladder

Other types of investigation include the following:

Nasendoscopy	The air passageway from the nostrils to the larynx
Mediastinoscopy	The tissues behind the breast bone or sternum to assess whether or not a lung cancer has spread to the lymph glands there
Colposcopy	The cervix ('neck of the womb')
Laparoscopy	The abdominal cavity

(leukaemia), or if the cancer is one of the few types that produce a characteristic chemical or 'tumour marker', which can be measured in the blood. These include some cancers of the prostate and testis and myeloma.

Nevertheless, blood tests can be useful in providing some information on your general state of health. Sometimes they can also suggest that a cancer may have spread to other organs such as the bones or liver. This is when the concentration of certain chemicals known as 'enzymes' normally released into the blood by these organs is above the normal range as a result of damage caused by the cancer. However, these tests are not foolproof – there are usually several possible causes of such abnormalities other than spread of the cancer.

X-RAYS AND SCANS

Often the first clear indication of the presence of a cancer is an abnormal appearance on an X-ray, for example, an abnormal shadow on a chest X-ray caused by a lung cancer occupying a space that would normally be filled largely with air. Tumours can also produce an abnormal breast X-ray (mammogram) and show up on a barium enema X-ray of the bowel.

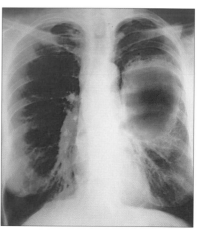

A mammogram is an X-ray picture of the breast taken with the breast compressed gently between two flat plates. Breast cancers can produce recognisable signs on the X-ray picture, particularly very small white flecks caused by small deposits of calcium within the cancerous tissue.

When barium is swallowed (barium meal or swallow) or inserted into the bowel via the rectum (barium enema), it shows up densely white on the X-ray, outlining the inner surface of the oesophagus, stomach or bowel. Normally the lining appears smooth but the presence of a cancer can cause it to appear irregular, or to bulge inwards indicating narrowing.

LUNG CANCER
This coloured chest X-ray shows a cancer in the left lung. The cancer is coloured red, and the normal lung tissue is shown as blue/green.

Sometimes other types of 'dye' or 'contrast medium', which show up white on an X-ray or scan, are injected into the bloodstream via a vein. For example, the blood may carry the dye to the kidney, which then excretes it into the urine. X-rays taken of the kidney and bladder (intravenous urogram [IVU] or pyelogram [IVP]) can then show up these organs quite clearly, and an abnormal appearance may suggest that a cancer is present.

You may need to have one of the various forms of scanning as part of the process of diagnosing cancer or assessing its extent. Computed tomography (CT) and magnetic resonance imaging (MRI) scans involve you having to lie still in what is usually a large doughnut-shaped structure. It will all be explained to you beforehand. CT scanning is very quick. MRI scanning takes somewhat longer, perhaps 15–20 minutes. These scanners can produce very impressive pictures of cross-sections or 'slices' of the part of the body being investigated, and they usually show growths much more clearly than simple X-rays. You may have to swallow or have an injection of a contrast medium, which will make the tumour or the nearby tissues show more clearly.

Ultrasound scanning is a process in which a probe is moved over the skin overlying the relevant part of the body. Occasionally it involves inserting a probe into the rectum or vagina. Images are produced on a screen by detecting very high-frequency, inaudible, 'sound' waves that are reflected off the internal tissues.

Isotope scanning is the creation of a picture by a 'gamma camera' that detects gamma rays emitted from

HAVING A CT SCAN
A CT scanner uses a series of X-ray beams to produce cross-sectional images (slices) of the body.

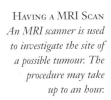

HAVING A MRI SCAN
An MRI scanner is used to investigate the site of a possible tumour. The procedure may take up to an hour.

the body after you have been injected with or swallowed a radioactive substance called an isotope. The most common type of isotope scan performed for cancer patients is a bone scan. The injected isotope is carried around the body by the bloodstream, but it tends to home in or 'concentrate' in any areas of bone where there is an attempt at healing any damage, which may have been caused by a tumour that has spread from another part of the body. The high concentration of isotope at such sites results in their appearance as 'hot spots' on the gamma camera picture of the skeleton. Interpretation can sometimes be difficult, however, and hot spots can often be caused by things other than cancer, such as degenerative disease ('wear and tear').

ISOTOPE SCAN
Before scanning, the patient swallows or is injected with a radioactive substance. This substance will concentrate in abnormal areas and appear as 'hot spots' on the gamma camera image.

As well as being used in the initial assessment of people suspected of or diagnosed as having cancer, X-rays and scans are used also to investigate symptoms that might possibly be caused by a recurrence in someone who has been treated for cancer in the past. However, it is important to realise that scans are not foolproof: even the most sensitive ones may fail to pick up a very small cancer and they quite often show suspicious abnormalities that turn out to be completely benign.

TUMOUR STAGING

Once a biopsy has confirmed the presence of a cancer it is common for it to be allocated to a certain 'stage'. This describes the size of the cancer and indicates whether or not there is evidence that it has invaded adjacent tissues or has spread via the lymphatic vessels to the lymph glands, or through the bloodstream to more distant sites. Various staging systems are in use but 'TNM' staging is the most widespread. 'T' refers to the primary tumour, 'N' to the lymph nodes and 'M' to distant spread (metastasis). A number is allocated to each letter. For example, a woman with a breast cancer three centimetres in diameter that has affected some of the lymph nodes in her armpit, but who does not have any evidence of more distant spread, could be said to have a 'T2N1M0' tumour. Here 'T2' indicates a primary tumour between two and five centimetres in diameter, 'N1' denotes involved but removable lymph nodes confined to the armpit, and 'M0' indicates that there has been no detectable distant spread.

Staging can be helpful in assessing prognosis, making recommendations for treatment and in assessing and comparing the results from treatment.

KEY POINTS

- You should always see your doctor promptly if you have any abnormal bleeding or an unexplained lump.

- Women over the age of 50 should take advantage of regular free NHS breast screening.

- Most cervical cancers can be cured, but almost 90 per cent of the few people who die from this disease have never had a routine smear.

- Analysis of a specimen of tissue under the microscope is essential for confirmation of a diagnosis of cancer.

- Scans are not foolproof.

Treatment in general

Once a diagnosis of cancer has been confirmed, and all other necessary investigations completed, the patient is then given advice by his or her doctor on what should happen next.
Priority is likely to be given to treatment directed against the cancer, but it is important that the overall plan for care takes account of physical symptoms, psychological well-being and family and other social circumstances.

There are three main types of treatment for cancer: surgery, radiotherapy and drugs. Overall, surgery is the single most effective treatment in curing cancer, but different types of cancer are treated in very different ways. Both radiotherapy and chemotherapy have the ability to destroy cancers while leaving the surrounding normal tissues completely intact. However, some cancers do not respond well to radiotherapy or drugs and are best treated by surgery. Others may be difficult or impossible to remove by an operation, but may respond well to other treatment.

When a cancer can be treated surgically, there is often no alternative treatment worth considering. However, radiotherapy may be equally or even more effective for

GETTING ADVICE
If you have been diagnosed with cancer, your consultant will discuss with you and your family the necessary steps to take to treat your particular condition.

some people with certain types of cancer, for example, some of those arising in the head and neck region or cervix. In such circumstances, radiotherapy may be the best option because it is not disfiguring, does not affect important functions such as the ability to speak or to swallow, or sometimes merely because it is simpler.

For many patients the best chance of cure is achieved nowadays by combinations of treatments. Some patients have to be admitted to hospital, particularly for surgery and intensive drug treatments. However, many are able to have their treatment as outpatients. Patients need to know what their particular treatment is likely to involve and many find it helpful to understand the reasons for what is being recommended.

GETTING RID OF CANCER
This is a basal cell carcinoma photographed before (top) and after (bottom) radiotherapy treatment, which has healed without scarring. This type of skin cancer responds well to radiotherapy.

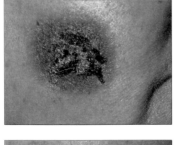

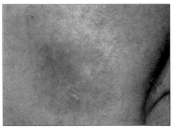

THE AIM OF TREATMENT

Whenever possible the goal of treatment is to eradicate the cancer completely, and this is now a realistic prospect for more and more people. This is partly because cancer is now often diagnosed at a relatively early stage, but partly also because treatments have improved. If your cancer has not spread from its original site, the outlook is often excellent.

However, some cancers have already obviously spread widely by the time they are first discovered, while others that appear localised have in fact spread to form undetectable microscopic metastases. In general, the outlook for patients with these cancers is less favourable, but nevertheless cure is now possible for a growing minority. These include those whose cancer is of a type that responds very well indeed to drug treatment, such as Hodgkin's disease and testicular tumours, and also those who have microscopic spread from other cancers that are often sensitive to drug treatment, such as breast cancer.

Treatment aimed at cure is quite often called 'radical'. Treatment aimed at relieving symptoms or prolonging life may be described as 'palliative'. Anti-cancer treatments can often provide excellent palliation. When used in this way, they are usually substantially less intensive or 'aggressive' than radical treatments, and as a result they are generally much better tolerated.

When aiming for cure, a high risk of troublesome side-effects may be acceptable. However, when cure is not possible there may be little justification for a powerful treatment if there is a significant chance that its side-effects will be at least as troublesome as the symptoms for which it is being offered. It is for this reason that the aim of treatment should be clear at the outset. However, just because a treatment is palliative this does not mean that it cannot have a powerful effect against the cancer. Indeed, some people lead normal lives with their cancers shrunken and under control for many years as a result of palliative treatment.

It is important that symptoms are dealt with as well, while anti-cancer treatment of one sort or another is being considered or given. These treatments may not deal satisfactorily with some symptoms, or they may be slow to work. Fortunately, there are very many other ways of relieving symptoms that may be used in addition to anti-cancer treatment, and sometimes instead of it. Often quite simple measures will suffice, but some patients require rather more help and support. This can often be provided very well by their general practitioners, the hospital doctors treating their cancer and the nurses who assist them, but some patients benefit greatly from more specialised symptom-relieving care. Increasing numbers of doctors and nurses now specialise in what is called 'palliative medicine' and provide care in patients' homes, in hospitals and in hospices (see Further Care, p.85). The growth in palliative medicine and in hospice-based care in recent years has been an enormous contribution to the improvement in quality of life for people with cancer, particularly those with more advanced or incurable disease. However, it should not be forgotten that palliative care can also help some whose cancer is curable: it should be available for anyone who has persistent troublesome symptoms, whatever the cause.

THE RIGHT TREATMENT

When planning and discussing your treatment with you, your doctor will want to be sure that it is tailored to your individual needs. There can be vast variation from one cancer to another in terms of how it looks under the microscope, its size, extent and behaviour. However, treatment for cancer needs to take into account not only the cancer, but the individual patient. No two people with cancer are exactly alike, physically or psychologically. Social circumstances may also be very relevant. Many aspects usually need to be considered before a decision is made about treatment.

Nevertheless, many patients fall into certain categories for which treatment is fairly uniform. In recent years, there has been a welcome trend towards increased standardisation of treatment. This helps to ensure that patients receive treatment that is widely considered to be appropriate by experts on their type of cancer. There are now frequent 'consensus development conferences' at which the latest research findings are discussed. These lead to publication of 'guidelines' that attempt to define good treatment policies for patients with certain types of cancer, and which have played a major role in eliminating undesirable variations in the quality of care.

All cancer treatments have side-effects. These may be minimal, for example, those from minor operations, regimens of low-dose radiotherapy and some drugs that may cause no upset at all. You may well be able to continue working and to lead a normal or near-normal life while you are having courses of radiotherapy and chemotherapy. At the other end of the spectrum are some very major operations or highly intensive radiotherapy or drug treatments, which can themselves make people very ill and which may even carry a small risk of death.

The treatment you are recommended to have will depend largely on the nature, position and extent of your cancer, but it is important that careful consideration is given to the risks and potential benefits of treatment for each individual patient.

If you are otherwise healthy and feeling robust, you will probably be willing to accept a high chance of troublesome side-effects from a treatment that offers a good chance of cure. In fact, the majority of those people with very serious tumours are prepared to undergo fairly unpleasant treatments for only a small chance of cure or a small improvement in the chance of cure. However, if there is realistically no prospect of cure the possible advantages and disadvantages of palliative treatment will need to be considered. Your age and general health may be important factors – you are likely to cope much better with treatment if you are otherwise fit than if you are relatively frail.

It may seem surprising, but the best option for some people is to have no treatment directed specifically against their cancer. Sometimes the treatments available do not work very well on their particular cancer or are more likely to do harm than good. In other cases it may be because the cancer is a 'mild' type that may grow only very slowly or even not at all over several years, and which may have little or no impact on quantity or quality of life.

COMBINING TREATMENTS

The careful use of combinations of different types of treatments is another reason for the improved results of recent years. In particular, drug treatments and radiotherapy are being given more often in addition to surgery, with the aim of eradicating any microscopic traces of cancer not removed by the operation. Surgery may fail to remove a cancer completely either because there are cancer cells left behind at the operation site, or because of metastases. If the amount of residual cancer is indeed of only microscopic proportions, then there may be quite a good chance that it can be eradicated completely by further treatment with radiotherapy or drugs or even both. Radiotherapy, being a local treatment, has only a local effect, whereas drugs have the potential to act throughout the body. Some patients with cancers for which the main treatment is radiotherapy will also benefit from additional treatment with drugs.

The use of additional radiotherapy or chemotherapy in this way is known as 'adjuvant' treatment. On occasions it is given before surgery, sometimes with the aim of making an operation possible or easier. For example, some women with fairly large breast cancers may be given drugs that shrink the tumour sufficiently to enable the surgeon to remove it without taking away the whole breast. Similarly, a course of radiotherapy beforehand may make it possible for a surgeon to remove a large and otherwise inoperable rectal cancer.

CANCER SERVICES

You may well be able to have your treatment at a cancer unit in your local district hospital, particularly if you are having surgery or chemotherapy. However, you may need to travel to a cancer centre further away from home if you need radiotherapy, more specialised surgery or intensive chemotherapy. Modern radiotherapy requires very expensive equipment and specially trained staff, so it makes sense to concentrate facilities in cancer centres in large towns or cities. Some surgical and drug treatments require equally specialised techniques and expertise. Thus, you may have to travel considerable distances for treatment, but this is usually worthwhile. You may be reassured to know that you are being cared for by staff who are experienced in treating your particular condition, especially if you have a less common type of cancer.

There is good evidence that treatment tends to be more successful if it is supervised or given by doctors who specialise in treating particular cancers. Most cancer surgery is now undertaken by surgeons who have special expertise in particular operations. The same philosophy applies to the non-surgical doctors who treat cancer patients, and to nursing and other 'paramedical' staff.

HOSPITAL SPECIALISTS

In addition to surgeons, the following types of specialist doctors are frequently involved in the care of patients with cancer during their hospital stay or visit.

- **Oncologist** Any doctor who specialises in cancer treatment, but usually, in practice, a doctor who supervises treatments with radiotherapy or drugs. Clinical oncologists specialise in both drug treatments and radiotherapy; medical oncologists specialise purely in drug treatments.
- **Haematologist** A doctor who specialises in abnormalities of the blood who will supervise your treatment if you have leukaemia and possibly if you have lymphoma or myeloma.
- **Palliative Care Physician** A doctor who specialises in the control of symptoms, particularly those resulting from more advanced cancers.

You may well be cared for by two or more specialists who will work together to decide the best treatment for you. It is now increasingly common for specialists to hold regular meetings to discuss individual patients. Ideally, most patients undergoing surgery for cancer should have an opinion from an oncologist. You have the right to ask for this if it is not offered.

Although it is usually doctors from one or more of the above categories that supervise the care of cancer patients, other specialists are also involved.

- **Pathologist** A doctor who examines tissue under the microscope and who confirms and categorises cancers.
- **Radiologist** A doctor who arranges and interprets X-rays and scans and may sometimes undertake some specialised surgical biopsies or treatments that have to be done under X-ray or scan supervision.

THE MEDICAL HIERARCHY

The titles of the medical staff who treat you in hospital may appear confusing at first. The list below will help to distinguish between the various doctors that you may see at hospital.

- **Consultant** A specialist – a senior hospital doctor who holds the ultimate responsibility for your care, but who is unlikely to be involved personally in every aspect. However, he or she will regularly hold outpatient clinics and 'ward rounds' to see new patients and to review the progress of those under their care. You can ask to see your consultant if you need to discuss something in particular.
- **Associate Specialist** A specialist who has trained to a high level but who does not hold the ultimate responsibility of a consultant.
- **Registrar** A doctor who is training to be a consultant. He or she may have very considerable experience and be expecting to become a consultant before long. Registrars supervise much of the day-to-day care on wards but also work in outpatient clinics. Surgical registrars frequently undertake operations or assist in them, depending on their seniority.
- **House Officer** Junior and senior house officers (SHOs) are fairly recently qualified doctors who are concerned largely with providing care on the wards.
- **Clinical Assistant, Staff Grade Doctor, Hospital Practitioner** Other doctors of variable experience who are not training to become consultants but who provide valuable assistance in various aspects of hospital care.

YOUR GENERAL PRACTITIONER

He or she may well know you and your family well and will continue to be responsible for coordinating much of your overall care, particularly that provided at home. You will have been referred to the hospital consultant in the first instance by your GP, and he or she will provide or arrange supportive care, both during and after treatment and at any other stage, as required. Your GP will also see you if you have any other illnesses while your cancer is being treated, and is able to provide help or advice with psychological or social problems. The doctors in the hospital will keep your doctor informed about your hospital treatment and progress. Although your cancer treatment is given in the hospital, your GP remains of great importance in your overall care.

PARAMEDICAL STAFF

A variety of other staff may be involved in your care, both in hospital (either as an out-patient or during your stay on a ward) and also at home.

● **Clinical Nurse Specialists** These may play an extremely important part in your care, both in hospital and at home. For example, oncology or chemotherapy nurses may give you your chemotherapy, while breast care and stoma care nurses are an essential part of the team caring for people with breast and bowel cancer. They can give a lot of practical advice and for many patients they become an important point of contact with the hospital.

● **Community Nurses** These provide care in your home, and include district nurses, practice nurses and health visitors.

● **Macmillan and Palliative Care Nurses** These give expert advice on symptom control and provide emotional support at home, hospital or the hospice.

● **Therapeutic Radiographers** These are specially trained to give the radiotherapy that has been prescribed by oncologists. They have a broad training in oncology and provide or arrange some supportive care as well.

You may also come into contact with other health professionals, such as physiotherapists, occupational therapists and dietitians during rehabilitation after your treatment. Medical social workers can offer practical advice and may help to arrange financial assistance and social support (for example, meals on wheels or help with housework), nursing or residential home accommodation.

DEALING WITH DOCTORS

You may well feel nervous and unsure of yourself when you have to see a doctor to discuss your condition, but it is important for you to talk as well as listen. Pressure of work, unfortunately, may mean that the specialist has less time to give to any one individual than he or she ideally would like, so you need to make the best use of the time available.

The specialist usually needs to know about any current symptoms, your general health and past medical history, and any particular concerns you may have about any aspect of the cancer or its treatment. You should also mention any psychological or social concerns relating to your illness. It is a good idea to take details of any medicines you are currently taking to the consultation (or the actual bottles or packs), to ensure that the specialist has accurate information.

As explained earlier, decisions about your treatment will be tailored to you as an individual, and the doctor may well need to know your feelings before recommending a particular course of action. First or early consultations are especially important as this is when investigations, their results, the diagnosis and the implications for treatment are discussed. You should take the opportunity to raise any worries you may have and to ask about what is on your mind. If necessary, write down a list of the questions you want to ask or points you want to raise, to use as a memory prompt. If you do not understand something the doctor says, do not be shy about asking for an explanation.

People differ as to the amount they want to know and the extent to which they want to be involved in decision-making. You may be one of those who prefers to accept explanations and treatment recommendations on trust without asking about them in any detail. However, if you do want more involvement, say so. The doctor will be happy to explain what the recommended treatment will involve, its chance of success, what its side-effects are likely to be and how it might be expected to affect your work or lifestyle. You can also ask about any possible alternatives.

Some people prefer to leave questions about the long-term outlook unasked for the time being, whereas others will want detailed statistical information at the outset. Everyone is different. All doctors recognise this and most will try to respond to your personal needs, but they cannot do this unless you make it clear what you want to know and, on occasions, what you do not want to know.

It can often be difficult to remember everything that is said by a specialist during a consultation. It is usually helpful to take along your husband, wife or someone else close to you – two memories are better than one. It is usually best to raise important questions or concerns earlier on, rather than leave them until the very end. Some patients also find it helpful to make brief notes during the consultation. Others have found it useful to tape record the consultation, although permission should always be asked for this as some doctors may find this somewhat 'off-putting' and disruptive to 'natural' conversation.

═══ PROGRESS REPORTS ═══

If you are seeing your doctor to discuss the progress of your treatment, it is helpful if you understand some of the words often used to describe how things are going.

• **Response** 'Response' is the term used to describe shrinkage of a cancer after treatment or at some stage during a course of treatment. Usually a cancer has to shrink quite significantly for this term to be used. A response may be defined as complete, when there is no evidence of any cancer remaining, or partial.

• **Remission** The term 'remission' may be used to describe a situation where the cancer has been greatly reduced and does not seem to be active, but has not disappeared. This is usually as a result of treatment but some cancers can occasionally go into remission of their own accord.

• **Recurrence or relapse** A 'recurrence' or 'relapse' is regrowth of a cancer after treatment that had previously been successful in controlling the disease. Recurrences are sometimes described as 'local' or 'distant', according to whether the problem is with the original tumour or because it has metastasised. Further treatment against the cancer is quite often recommended following a recurrence, especially if a cure still seems feasible, but in other situations this may not necessarily be in the patient's best overall interest. Much depends on the particular circumstances.

TAKING IT ALL IN
It may be difficult to remember everything that is said during a consultation. Some patients tape record their conversation with the specialist (with his or her permission) so that they may go over it again at home.

49

SECOND OPINIONS

You have the right to ask for a second opinion and this is normally arranged by your GP, sometimes after discussion with the specialist to whom you have been referred. Specialists looking after people with cancer understand full well why you may want to do this and are likely to support your request. Sometimes, particularly in complicated or difficult cases, they may suggest a second opinion themselves.

It is usually important that a second opinion is given fairly quickly, particularly if there is a need for prompt treatment. It is also important that the second opinion is sought from someone who has the appropriate experience and expertise and that he or she is provided with all the relevant information. However, you should realise that a second opinion that is different from the first is not necessarily a better one.

CONSENT TO TREATMENT

You may be asked to sign a consent form before treatment. This goes hand in hand with ensuring that you have all the information you need about the possible risks of treatment, either verbally or in written form. This is done partly to protect you from agreeing to a treatment through ignorance of any risks involved, but also partly to protect the hospital from legal action in the event of anything going wrong despite competent care.

Patients should bear in mind the fact that all medical treatments have side-effects in some people. You may well become worried if you are presented with a list of possible adverse effects without realising that the actual chance of a severe side-effect occurring is often very low. However, some anti-cancer treatments are more powerful than others and some have greater potential for doing harm. Thus some patients in some situations may find it helpful, with the help and advice of their doctor, to try to weigh up the relative chances of benefit and of harm (the 'risk–benefit ratio').

For the great majority of anti-cancer treatments, this ratio is substantially in your favour, but there is also no doubt that there are some possible treatments that, in certain situations, stand a rather greater chance of doing more harm than good. It is important that you have as much realistic information as you want about the potential risks and benefits of any treatment before agreeing to it, whether or not you are asked to sign a consent form.

KEY POINTS

- Cancer treatment has become increasingly standardised, but individual circumstances remain very important.

- Your GP will play a very important part in your overall care.

- Some people will need to travel some way to get the best available treatment.

- It is worth taking some trouble to prepare yourself before consultation.

- Consultations are opportunities for two-way communication.

Surgery

If your doctor has reason to suspect that you may have cancer, you are likely to be referred initially to a surgeon. This is partly because some kind of surgical procedure is very often required to make a definitive diagnosis, and partly because surgery is the best treatment or the best initial treatment for many types of cancer.

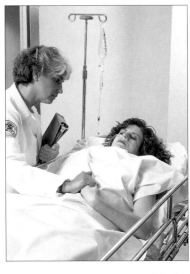

HAVING SURGERY
Any type of surgery is likely to make a patient apprehensive, but the great majority of operations proceed according to plan.

Where cancer is discovered, its extent may also be established during an operation; and this is sometimes an important aim of the procedure. Examples include armpit lymph node removal ('axillary dissection' or 'clearance') for women who are undergoing surgery for breast cancer, and a thorough inspection of the abdominal cavity (during a 'staging laparotomy') for women who are undergoing removal of ovarian cancer.

It is only understandable that most people will feel nervous about having to have an operation. However, most cancer operations proceed very well. It is, of course, inevitable that the results are not always perfect, but it is not feasible to discuss in detail here the possible short- or long-term adverse effects of particular operations, which may vary from relatively minor procedures lasting a few minutes to major undertakings over many hours.

Some operations do, of course, leave substantial long-term effects on appearance, function or both. Other operations carry risks of certain side-effects for some patients, for example arm swelling ('lymphoedema' – see p.99) after axillary clearance and impotence after surgery

Surgical Terms

A range of special terms is used to refer to surgical procedures, and some of these are encountered in the context of cancer treatment. These are the principal ones:

RESECTION — The removal of a tumour or organ; words ending in '-ectomy' mean the same thing. For example, removal of a lung lobe containing a cancer may be called a 'pulmonary lobectomy' and removal of a cancer-containing prostate gland a 'prostatectomy'.

RADICAL — In addition to cutting out the obvious tumour, this involves the removal of tissue near or connected to the tumour or organ involved, with the aim of doing everything possible to get rid of every last cancer cell.

WORDS ENDING IN '-OSTOMY' — When one of the body's internal tubes is blocked by a tumour or when part of it has to be removed, the surgeon may need to bypass the obstruction and create an inlet or outlet by joining the tube to an artificial opening made in the skin (a 'stoma': see below). For example, joining the windpipe or trachea to the overlying skin is called a 'tracheostomy' and may be temporary or permanent, depending on the circumstances. Joining the large bowel or colon to a stoma in the abdominal skin is called a 'colostomy'. This too may be temporary or permanent.

STOMA — An artificial opening in the skin to allow the contents of the underlying tube to exit the body. After a colostomy, for example, a bag will be fitted over the stoma to collect the bowel contents. Modern designs enable the great majority of people who undergo this procedure to lead virtually normal lives.

53

for rectal or prostate cancer. Any such risks will normally be discussed in detail with you beforehand, but if you feel you need more information do not be afraid to ask for it. Some patients only need to spend a very short time in hospital afterwards, others two or three weeks or even longer. Some are able to return to a normal lifestyle almost straightaway, whereas others may take some months to recover fully after major operations. Although most patients will feel some discomfort in the period immediately after the operation, they can nevertheless expect to receive a high standard of postoperative care nowadays. including very good pain control.

SURGERY FOR CURE

In most cases, the surest way of eradicating a localised cancer is, where possible, to excise it (cut it out) with an adequate margin of surrounding normal tissue. Surgery cannot cure a cancer that has spread to distant parts of the body or when it is not technically possible to remove the cancer completely.

Most cancer surgery is conducted as a carefully planned or 'cold' procedure, the diagnosis having already been made with near or absolute certainty. However, a small minority of people are first discovered to have cancer during an emergency operation made necessary by complications of the cancer, such as perforation or obstruction of the bowel. In this situation, the results of surgery unfortunately tend to be rather less good. This is because these tumours are quite often at an advanced stage and also because the person concerned may not be in good general health.

There has been a trend in recent decades towards less radical surgery for some tumours. For example, providing the size and position of the growth are favourable, it may be possible to remove a cancer from a woman's breast, together with sufficient surrounding tissue ('wide local excision'), while avoiding the need to remove the whole breast (mastectomy). This type of operation is then followed up with radiotherapy to the breast to get rid of any remaining microscopic traces of cancer, and the prospects for cure are just as good as with mastectomy. A similar combination of less aggressive surgery and radiotherapy can also be used to treat the much rarer soft tissue sarcomas.

In other situations, however, surgery is more extensive than it used to be. For example, most women with breast cancer now have lymph nodes removed from under their arms, in addition to surgery to the breast itself. This is quite often a thorough removal of all the nodes that can be identified, known as an 'axillary clearance'. Not only can such procedures eradicate any metastases that might be present in the nodes, they can also give useful information about whether or not the cancer is likely to have spread microscopically to other parts of the body. The risk of this increases if there has been spread to the lymph nodes. This knowledge may be used to advise patients about what further treatment they should have. Some women who have lymph node metastases from breast cancer will have their chance of cure increased significantly by chemotherapy or hormonal treatment.

Surgery has long been known as a potential cure for many people whose cancer has spread to nearby lymph nodes, but there is now growing enthusiasm for surgery for carefully selected individuals whose cancer has spread via the bloodstream to a fairly small and removable part of the lung or liver. The chance of success tends to be

Different Types of Breast Surgery

The nature of surgery carried out in breast cancer depends on the size and position of the tumour. It is often possible to remove a cancerous tumour from the breast without carrying out a mastectomy.

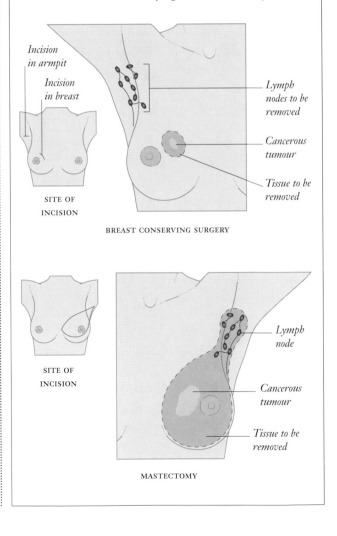

Incision in armpit

Incision in breast

SITE OF INCISION

Lymph nodes to be removed

Cancerous tumour

Tissue to be removed

BREAST CONSERVING SURGERY

SITE OF INCISION

Lymph node

Cancerous tumour

Tissue to be removed

MASTECTOMY

greater when there is a long interval between treatment of the primary growth and the development of a metastasis.

RECONSTRUCTIVE SURGERY

Considerable progress has also been made in restoring appearance or function after operations to remove cancer. For example, many women who have had a breast removed are now offered surgery to create a 'new' breast, either by inserting some form of artificial 'implant' beneath the muscle underlying the skin, or by building up a new 'breast' using muscle and fatty tissue (a 'flap') from the back or lower abdominal wall. The results, although not perfect, are frequently highly satisfactory. They can make a huge psychological difference for those women who understandably find it very difficult to live with the loss of a breast.

Such reconstructive procedures often involve highly specialised surgical expertise. This is sometimes provided by plastic surgeons. As well as contributing to the care of some patients with breast cancer, they perform a very important role also in helping to restore appearance and function after major surgery for cancers involving the mouth and throat and other nearby structures.

Some reconstructive procedures are done at the time of tumour removal, with the plastic surgeon operating together with the surgeon who removes the tumour. Others may be done some time later.

The artificial material that is used in any form of reconstructive surgery is known as a 'prosthesis'. Some people with bone sarcomas of the limbs can now benefit from bone replacement prosthetic surgery after removal of the growth, thereby avoiding the need to amputate the limb concerned.

Preventing Fractures

Sometimes cancers spread via the bloodstream to the bones. When this occurs, the affected bone may become weak and may even fracture. To prevent a fracture, sometimes the bone may be pinned using a metal rod.

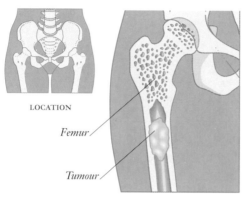

LOCATION

Femur

Tumour

BEFORE SURGERY

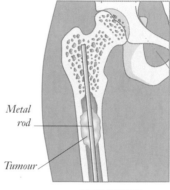

Metal rod

Tumour

AFTER SURGERY

PALLIATIVE SURGERY

Surgical procedures are also performed to relieve symptoms. Sometimes this is in conjunction with other treatments aimed at destroying the cancer.

Prosthetic tubes or 'stents' may be inserted to relieve obstruction caused by a growth. This is often done for people with cancer of the oesophagus. Obstructions within the abdomen are sometimes relieved by 'by-pass' operations. Metal prostheses may be inserted into a bone that has been fractured or substantially weakened by a metastatic tumour. This restores strength to the bone and allows a rapid return of normal or near-normal use to the limb. Lasers are sometimes used to bore a hole through tumours obstructing the oesophagus or one of the major air tubes or 'bronchi' within the lung. A tracheostomy may be necessary when a tumour is obstructing the voice box or larynx and causing difficulty in breathing.

A tumour that is pressing on the spinal cord can cause leg weakness by interfering with the nerve supply to the muscles. This can sometimes be relieved by partial removal of the tumour by a neurosurgeon or orthopaedic surgeon. Some people with breast and prostate cancers benefit from surgical removal of their ovaries or testes, operations known respectively as 'oophorectomy' and 'orchidectomy'. These cancers are often susceptible to hormonal influences, so removing the sources of these hormones can bring about marked tumour shrinkage that may last for a long time. Finally, surgical procedures are also undertaken occasionally to control bleeding from a growth.

KEY POINTS

- Confirmation of a diagnosis of cancer is usually established by some form of surgical procedure.
- Surgery cures more cancers than any other treatment used alone.

Radiotherapy

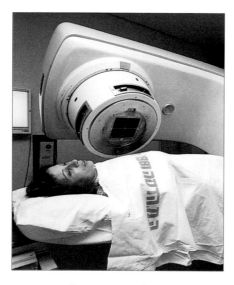

Most radiotherapy is given using beams of high-energy X-rays, much more powerful than those used for taking ordinary 'X-rays'. The X-rays used in radiotherapy are also administered in much longer bursts – for example, a minute or so, compared with less than a second for diagnostic pictures. These beams shed their energy into the cells of the tissues through which they pass.

RADIOTHERAPY
During treatment, the patient must lie completely still while the beam of radiation is focused on the target area.

You will have to lie still while you are undergoing radiotherapy, but you do not feel anything, and from your point of view the only difference from having an ordinary X-ray is that radiotherapy lasts longer. You do not become radioactive.

THE TARGET

Radiotherapy targets the DNA in the nucleus of the cell because, if this is damaged sufficiently, cells will lose their ability to replicate. If cells in a cancer that die naturally are not being replaced by new ones, not only will the cancer stop growing, it will become smaller and will eventually wither away and disappear altogether.

Normal cells are affected to some extent by radiotherapy too. Fortunately, normal cells in general have a greater ability to repair radiation damage than cancer cells. The therapy is done in such a way as to ensure that cancer cells receive the highest dose of radiation while minimising, as far as possible, the amount that reaches nearby normal cells. This may be done by using crossed beams focused on the tumour or by shielding some of the normal tissue (see below).

HOW CANCERS RESPOND

Cancers vary considerably in their sensitivity to radiotherapy: some types are more likely to be totally eradicated than others. How quickly they respond to treatment is also very variable. Some cancers will continue to shrink slowly and eventually disappear long after a course of radiotherapy has been completed, possibly over many weeks. Others will respond much more quickly, particularly those in which the cells were dividing rapidly before treatment.

In general, smaller cancers have a greater chance of being completely destroyed by radiotherapy than larger ones. This is partly because of the sheer volume of tissue involved, but also because larger tumours tend to outgrow the blood vessels supplying them, resulting in a reduced blood supply and thus less oxygen at their centre. Oxygen is very important to the process of DNA damage caused by radiation. Oxygen is carried to the tissues by the red blood cells, so if the tumour has a poor blood supply, or if there is a lowered concentration of red cells in the blood (anaemia), radiotherapy may be less effective.

Another reason why radiotherapy may sometimes not achieve complete tumour destruction is that the tumour cells continue to replicate rapidly in between daily treatments. One way of trying to deal with this that is occasionally used in certain situations, is to give radiotherapy two or three times per day in a very short and intensive course of treatment. This is known as 'hyperfractionated' and 'accelerated' treatment.

Radiotherapy can destroy a cancer only if it is possible to target the beams so that they encompass the whole of the tumour. It can be used to treat rather larger portions of tissue than can often be dealt with by surgery, but is nevertheless a fairly localised form of treatment. Another crucial factor is the 'dose' of radiotherapy, measured in units called 'grays'. Some cancers will respond well to relatively low doses whereas others may need very high doses if they are to be destroyed.

Radiotherapy is usually given in quite high dosage (radical radiotherapy) when it is given by itself with the intent of completely destroying a cancer. A slightly lower dose is given when radiotherapy is being given as adjuvant (aiding) treatment to prevent a cancer returning after surgical removal. The dosage is usually considerably lower when the treatment is palliative. In this situation the aim is to cause sufficient tumour shrinkage to alleviate symptoms, but not to eradicate the cancer completely.

SIDE-EFFECTS OF RADIOTHERAPY

If you are receiving low-dosage radiotherapy you may not notice any side-effects whatsoever, but those receiving high-dose treatment can usually expect to experience them. What they are, and their severity, depend on the part and amount of the body being treated, the dose of radiotherapy and also on how sensitive a particular individual is to treatment.

The most common side-effects occur during or immediately after treatment and are short lasting, when they are described as being 'acute'. They usually disappear quite quickly after treatment. A few people may develop so-called 'late' side-effects, which do not become apparent until several months or even sometimes several years after treatment. These effects can be long lasting ('chronic') or even permanent. It is unusual for long-lasting effects to be particularly troublesome, but small risks are often justifiable when aiming for cure.

SHORT-TERM EFFECTS

The normal tissues that tend to be most sensitive to radiotherapy in the short term are those where the cells are normally dividing quite rapidly to replace those lost by wear and tear. These include the skin and the membranes lining the mouth, throat, oesophagus, bowel and bladder. Inflammation, soreness, diarrhoea and urinary frequency are thus quite common side-effects, depending on the part of the body being treated. Some patients who undergo radiotherapy will get skin soreness rather like sunburn but, unless a superficial tumour is being treated, it is now unusual for this to be severe, as modern radiotherapy beams can deliver the maximum dose deep to the surface.

Other quite common acute side-effects include tiredness, nausea (particularly if the upper abdomen is being irradiated) and hair loss if treatment beams go through the scalp. This is not usually permanent, although there may be patches where the hair does not regrow if radiotherapy is being given in fairly high dosage for a brain tumour. Bone marrow, the blood cell factory, is also very sensitive to radiation but this is usually only a problem in the unusual event of treatment being given to a large part of the body containing a large proportion of the total amount of marrow.

Before having radiotherapy you will be warned about the more common side-effects and probably given advice about how, for example, to care for your skin or change your diet to try to prevent the reaction becoming at all severe. If your abdomen or pelvis is being treated, you may be recommended to cut out high-fibre foods, including fruit and green vegetables, until the reaction has settled. This is because they can make diarrhoea worse. If necessary, you may be given one of the various medications available to lessen side-effects. Occasionally, it is necessary to interrupt the course of treatment for a week or so to allow side-effects to settle.

Tiredness and other acute side-effects of treatment can sometimes interfere significantly with normal living, but many people have only slight side-effects. You may feel well enough to continue working during your treatment and your doctor may encourage you to do so if you feel up to it. However, it is sensible to take things easy if you feel tired or unable to carry on with your normal life.

LONG-TERM EFFECTS

Tissues that tend to be sensitive to radiotherapy in the longer term include the lungs, kidneys, the eye lenses (where cataracts may form) and the testes and ovaries (possibly resulting in infertility). However, significant damage to these tissues can usually be avoided by careful treatment planning.

Other rare long-term effects include lymphoedema (see p.99) as a result of treatment to the armpit after surgery for breast cancer, and bowel damage following radiotherapy for cancer of the cervix. Radiotherapy can cause mouth dryness if the salivary glands are being treated, and this can predispose to both tooth decay and gum disease. Patients at risk for this problem should have a specialist dental assessment before treatment and be given advice about caring for their teeth in the future.

Growing tissues are also very sensitive to radiotherapy and this has important implications for treatment for children. Finally, there is a theoretical long-term risk that another cancer might be caused many years later by the radiation. In practice, however, the chance of this happening is extremely low.

EXTERNAL RADIOTHERAPY

Radiotherapy is usually given to a fairly localised part of the body. It is given mostly using high-energy, deeply penetrating, 'megavoltage' X-ray beams produced in large machines called linear accelerators. Sometimes, less penetrating, lower-energy 'orthovoltage' beams produced by much smaller machines are used to treat relatively superficial growths, particularly skin cancers. Electron beams produced in linear accelerators are also used sometimes to treat fairly superficial tissues. All these methods involve beams of radiation being 'shone' into the body from outside, and are known sometimes as 'external' radiotherapy.

External radiotherapy is given in a 'treatment room', which has specially thick walls, to prevent radiation escaping from it. The treatment machine is controlled by radiographers. They stay outside the room while they administer treatment. If they remained inside with the patient they would receive, over time, a significant cumulative dose from 'scattered' radiation.

PLANNING TREATMENT

Radiotherapy can vary enormously in complexity. Some treatments are technically quite simple. When treating skin cancers, or sometimes when giving radiotherapy to relieve a symptom, the oncologist merely has to draw on the skin to indicate the area requiring treatment, and then specify the dose, the number of treatments and their frequency.

At the other end of the spectrum, treatments can become very complex, using at least two and sometimes several radiation beams, which enter the body from different angles and converge at the site of the cancer. The aim is to give this part of the body a high dose in comparison to that given to the adjacent normal tissues. Meticulous planning is required, and you may have to have CT or MRI scans to define as accurately as possible the position, size and shape of the part of the body to be treated. Computers are then used to work out how best to arrange the treatment beams so that they will deliver the required dose to the intended target, while keeping the dose to the surrounding normal structures to a minimum. Sometimes the beams will be shaped specially to achieve this. Once the oncologist has checked the resulting 'treatment plan' and prescribed the treatment, radiotherapy can then begin.

To be certain that the treatment beams are entering the body at the correct positions, 'reference points' are often marked on the skin, either with felt-tip pens or as pinprick-sized tattoos. If felt-tip pen marks are used, you will be warned not to wash them off! Quite often a final accuracy check is made on a 'simulator' by taking X-rays corresponding to the treatment beams, or by producing precise pictures of the tissue being irradiated on the radiotherapy machine itself.

As accuracy is so vital, you may be fitted with an 'immobilisation mould' or 'shell', sometimes also known as a 'jig', especially if you are having radiotherapy to the head or neck. This is an individualised transparent plastic mould that fits like a glove over the part of the body being treated, and which is fixed to the treatment couch, so stopping you moving even very slightly during treatment. An additional benefit is that the entry points of treatment beams can be marked on the plastic surface without resorting to skin tattoos.

How Long Is the Treatment?

Although most individual radiotherapy treatments take only a couple of minutes or less to deliver, all the position and other accuracy checks often mean that you are in the treatment room for 10–15 minutes per session.

Sometimes, particularly when the main aim of treatment is to relieve symptoms, only one or two sessions or 'fractions' are required. In other instances, treatment may continue once a day for up to six or seven weeks. For long courses such as this you will probably have the weekends off. However, occasionally a more intensive short programme may be preferred, involving 'continuous'. hyperfractionated and accelerated treatment ('CHART') two or three times per day, including over the weekend.

Treatment From the Inside

Some cancers are best treated by placing small amounts of a radioactive 'isotope' inside the patient, either within or very close to the growth. The isotope emits rays, known as 'gamma rays', which have identical properties to X-rays. This makes it possible to deliver a high radiation dose to the cancer cells, while normal tissues a little further away

Internal Radiation Treatment

Some cancers, such as those of the womb lining or cervix, may be treated by inserting radioactive sources inside the body very close to the cancer.

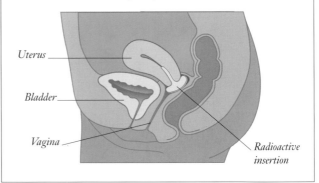

Uterus

Bladder

Vagina

Radioactive insertion

receive only a considerably reduced dose. This can decrease the chance of troublesome side-effects.

This method is used most often in the treatment of cancer of the cervix, when radioactive caesium is inserted into the uterine cavity and upper vagina and left there for many hours, or for a rather shorter time if a 'high-dose rate' technique is used. This type of treatment is known as 'intracavitary' treatment because the source of the radiotherapy is placed within a body cavity. It is quite often given in addition to a course of external treatment.

For other growths, for example, some breast and tongue cancers, small pieces of the isotope may be placed actually within the tumour. This is known as 'interstitial' treatment. Most intracavitary and interstitial treatments are now given using computer-controlled equipment that propels tiny isotope pellets by compressed air through hollow tubes, which the oncologist has inserted in the correct position while the patient was under an anaesthetic. Once in place in the cavity or inside the tumour, the pellets are left there for the required amount of time. They are then sucked back into the lead-lined safe in which they are stored safely.

In another type of radiotherapy, you may be given an injection of a radioactive isotope or asked to swallow it. It is then carried round the body in the bloodstream. The isotopes used in this form of treatment have a strong tendency to 'home in' on certain tissues such as benign or malignant thyroid tissue (radioactive iodine) and bone metastases from prostate cancer (radioactive strontium). These radioactive isotopes emit electrons (or 'beta rays') that have a very short range, but which can destroy cancer cells when released by the isotope very close to them. As the cell-killing effect is directed predominantly against the cancer cells, these treatments usually cause few side-effects.

KEY POINTS

- Radiotherapy, like surgery, is a localised form of treatment.
- Radiotherapy can potentiallly destroy a cancer completely while leaving the surrounding normal cells intact.
- You do not feel anything during treatment.
- Different cancers vary considerably in their sensitivity to radiotherapy.
- High-dose radiotherapy given for cure often carries a low risk of long-term side-effects, but this is a usually a risk worth taking.

Drug treatment

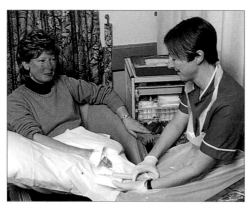

HAVING CHEMOTHERAPY
This patient is receiving chemotherapy, in which an anticancer drug is injected into the bloodstream in order to kill cancerous cells in any affected parts of the body.

Unlike surgery and radiotherapy, drug treatment is 'whole body' treatment. Anti-cancer drugs are carried by the bloodstream to almost every part of the body. Thus it is possible for drugs to kill cancer cells wherever they are. Drugs are particularly useful, therefore, in the treatment of cancers that have spread from the original tumour to other parts of the body, or when there is a significant chance that they may have done so even though this cannot be detected.

There are three reasons for giving anti-cancer drugs:
• To try to destroy the cancer by the drug treatment alone, aiming for a complete cure.
• To try to improve the chance of cure by eradicating any residual microscopic disease left behind after surgery or radiotherapy, or by shrinking the cancer sufficiently to make these treatments easier or more successful.
• To try to shrink the cancer sufficiently to achieve symptom improvement or prolongation of life.

There are two main categories of drugs that are used to treat cancer: cytotoxic and hormonal ('endocrine'). Cytotoxic (cell poisoning) drug treatment is commonly known as 'chemotherapy'. Chemotherapy often has a significant effect on normal cells as well as cancer cells, which potentially results in a variety of side-effects. In contrast, hormonal treatments are usually much 'gentler'. However, chemotherapy is active against a far wider range of cancers than hormonal treatment and it also tends to act rather more quickly. Different people with the same type of cancer will often respond very differently to the same treatment, whether hormonal or cytotoxic.

CHEMOTHERAPY

Chemotherapy works by interfering with 'mitosis' (cell division). Just like radiotherapy, if it is completely successful in stopping cancer cells dividing, the tumour will eventually disappear as its cells die of 'old age' without being replaced.

Cytotoxic chemotherapy, rather like radiotherapy, is particularly active against both cancer cells and normal cells that are dividing. When chemotherapy is successful, its effect is often seen most quickly in cancers where the cells were dividing rapidly beforehand. Similarly, the side-effects tend to be prominent in those tissues or organs where the normal cells are usually dividing quickly. These include the bone marrow where the blood cells are made, the hair follicles and the inner lining membrane of the bowel.

As with radiotherapy, giving chemotherapy involves trying to strike the right balance between killing cancer cells on the one hand, and avoiding intolerable side-effects on the other. Fortunately, considerable advances have been made in recent years in lessening the side-effects of chemotherapy, which are now much less troublesome than many people imagine. Indeed, some forms of chemotherapy now cause virtually no unpleasant symptoms whatsoever. Somewhat surprisingly, friends and relatives still occasionally lead patients to expect chemotherapy to be much more unpleasant than it really is.

As some medicines can interfere with chemotherapy, the oncologist responsible for your treatment should be made aware of all other medicines that you may be taking.

There are many different cytotoxic drugs and a vast number of combinations of them. They are used to treat a wide range of different cancers and in a variety of circumstances. Some types of cancer respond in general much better than others. Also, individual drugs vary considerably in how well they work against particular cancers. Although space here is too limited for a detailed description of chemotherapy for any particular cancer, you can obtain further information from some of the sources listed under Useful Addresses (see p.116).

COMBINING DRUGS

A proportion of the cells of any cancer is likely to be resistant to a particular individual drug, even if that drug is very effective against the remainder. This is why most chemotherapy involves taking combinations of drugs in the hope of lessening the chance of treatment failure because of resistance. Also, lower doses of individual drugs can be used in combinations than might be needed if they were being given singly, and this can sometimes lessen particular side-effects.

When prescribing 'combination chemotherapy', your doctor will aim to choose drugs that tend to be active against your particular cancer, but which have rather different side-effects. The chosen regimen may also incorporate drugs that interfere with different stages of cell division. However, the chosen combination will ultimately be based on its track record in treating large numbers of people with the same kind of cancer in the past.

HAVING CHEMOTHERAPY

Sometimes chemotherapy may be taken by mouth ('orally'), but more often it is given by injection into a vein ('intravenously' or 'IV'). Having a chemotherapy intravenous injection started usually feels just like having blood taken for a blood test. You might feel a coolness or other unusual sensation in the area of the injection.

You will probably have chemotherapy intermittently, say once every three weeks or twice a month, in the out-patient clinic. Usually it is given as a single injection or 'infusion' (using a 'drip') into a vein on the hand or lower arm over a few minutes or sometimes over several hours. Injections may be repeated daily for a few days, or the drug may be infused continuously over a day or a few days, with two- to three-week intervals between courses. There are very many different treatment schedules.

You may need to stay in hospital if you are having more intensive and toxic treatments. Infusional chemotherapy quite often requires you to be treated as an inpatient on the ward, although it is possible to administer some drugs by continuous infusion at home using a small pump strapped to the body. This method is used particularly for those patients who are treated by continuous infusion over prolonged periods.

If you need prolonged infusions or very frequent injections, you may have a 'central venous catheter' or 'line' inserted. These are thin flexible tubes that have their inner end positioned in a large vein inside the chest and the other end outside, so that drugs can be injected into it. The outer end may be on the front of the chest (Hickman or Groshong catheters) or in the arm in the case of 'peripherally inserted central catheters' ('PICC lines'), which are put in via an arm vein.

Sometimes the outer end of the catheter is not brought out through the skin, but is attached instead to an 'implantable port', a barely noticeable small container placed surgically just underneath the skin of the chest wall. Injections are then made through the skin into the port. These ports are not suitable for everyone, but those who do have them find that they do not interfere much with normal life. You have to be in hospital to have the catheter inserted, but you will then be able to go home once it is in place.

Each individual period of chemotherapy administration, whether given in a single injection or over a few days, is commonly known as a 'course', although sometimes single injections or infusions are called 'pulses'. Treatment should always be given by specially trained staff, and you will usually be treated by a highly qualified nurse.

HOW LONG DOES CHEMOTHERAPY LAST?

Just how long your chemotherapy treatment will continue depends on a number of factors. When given with the aim of cure or as an 'adjuvant' (aiding) treatment, there will probably be a clearly defined duration (provided of course there is no evidence that it is not working satisfactorily), based on past clinical experience and research. It may be as short as a couple of months or occasionally up to a year or even longer. When the aim is to relieve symptoms or prolong life, how long the treatment lasts depends very much on the effect of treatment on the cancer, and on any side-effects.

SIDE-EFFECTS

These days many people find that chemotherapy causes few serious problems and, although you will probably experience some side-effects, these are often not at all severe. They vary enormously according to the drugs and dosage used and your general health. There are, however, some side-effects that are quite common to a large number of drugs. The gaps in between treatment courses allow the normal cells to recover, particularly the bone marrow cells, which are generally more sensitive than other normal cells to chemotherapy.

● **Effects on the blood (and why blood counts have to be checked)** The bone marrow produces the different types of blood cells. The red cells carry oxygen around the body, the white cells fight infection and the platelets clot the blood to seal leakages in blood vessels. A deficiency of red blood cells is known as anaemia. 'Leucopenia' is a deficiency of white cells and a deficiency of platelets is called 'thrombocytopenia'.

Most cytotoxic drugs interfere temporarily with bone marrow function, particularly the production of white cells and platelets. Bone marrow toxicity is the most common and generally the most important side-effect of chemotherapy. The concentration ('level' or 'count') of the white cells and the platelets in the blood will usually fall during the week or so after chemotherapy, the extent depending on both the drug(s) used and the dosage.

Once leucopenia reaches a certain severity, you are at an increased risk of getting an infection and your immune system is less able to deal with it. For this reason, you will probably be advised to try to avoid close contact with people with infections, or with children who have recently received immunisation with a 'live' vaccine. You may also

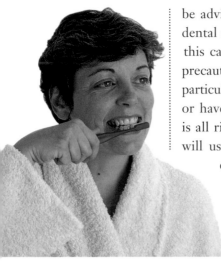

PERSONAL HYGIENE
Patients with a low white cell blood count should keep teeth and gums clean as they can harbour bacteria.

be advised to pay extra attention to personal hygiene, dental and skin care, and to avoid squeezing pimples as this can release bacteria into your bloodstream. Such precautions are especially important if you are receiving particularly intensive treatment. Patients who are having or have recently had chemotherapy should check if it is all right for them to have any immunisations. They will usually be advised to avoid 'live' vaccines (those containing living organisms).

If you are having chemotherapy, you should always tell your doctor immediately if you have any signs of an infection, particularly a fever, chills or sweating. If this happens, your blood count will usually be checked immediately. If your white cell count is below a certain level, you will probably have to have 'broad-spectrum' antibiotics intravenously. This will help your body's own immune system to fight off the infection, while waiting for the count to recover.

Very occasionally, thrombocytopenia becomes so severe that you start to bleed or bruise very easily and, again, you should report this to your doctor promptly. If necessary, you can then be given a transfusion of platelets from donated blood while waiting for your marrow to recover. If your platelet count is low, you must make every effort to avoid even the most minor injuries. Anaemia caused by chemotherapy is usually a much less urgent problem. However, it can cause skin pallor and symptoms such as weakness, tiredness and breathlessness.

Normally the blood counts recovers fairly rapidly, but it is important that it has returned to normal by the time you have your next course of treatment. If not, it is usually necessary to postpone further treatment until the count has recovered, and sometimes it is then decided to reduce the chemotherapy dosage. If further chemotherapy were to be given when the blood count was already low, there would be a greatly increased risk of serious complications occurring. This is why your blood count is checked routinely before each course or pulse of chemotherapy. Occasionally 'growth factor' (also known as 'colony-stimulating factor' or CSF) injections are given after chemotherapy to stimulate the recovery of the white cells, and similarly 'epoetin' for red cell recovery, although anaemia is usually readily correctable by a blood transfusion.

● **Sickness** Nausea and vomiting are well-known side-effects of chemotherapy, but they are now much less of a problem than they used to be. Several drugs cause this only to a slight degree, if at all. If you are taking drugs that cause more troublesome sickness, the problem can usually be prevented or greatly lessened by modern anti-dotes. Anti-sickness drugs (called 'antiemetics') are now often given routinely to stop symptoms developing, sometimes starting the day before the chemotherapy is given (see Nausea and vomiting on pp.100–101).

● **Hair loss** Another well-known and common side-effect is hair loss or 'alopecia', although not all drugs cause it. Hair is sensitive because the cells in the hair follicles divide rapidly. Sometimes alopecia is only slight, but with some drugs it becomes virtually total. Hair loss usually begins about two and a half weeks after the start of treatment. Hair always regrows once chemotherapy is completed, usually starting to do so about three weeks after the last course. You may find that at first your hair is curlier than before. Occasionally some regrowth occurs during chemotherapy. Hair loss can occur on all parts of

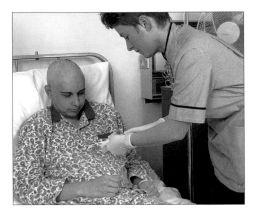

ALOPECIA
Hair loss, particularly on the head, is a common side-effect of chemotherapy. The hair usually begins to fall out about two and a half weeks after the start of treatment.

the body, but it most commonly affects the hair on the head.

Fortunately, society's attitude to hair loss has changed considerably in recent years, perhaps partly as a result of changing fashions and partly because we are all more used to seeing and reading about people who have lost their hair after cancer treatment. Although you may well be understandably upset at the thought of losing your hair, you will probably find that in reality you cope with it better than you expected.

If you are not happy to leave your head uncovered (although increasing numbers of people are), you should choose a wig or hair piece before your hair starts falling out. It is usually a good idea to shave off your remaining hair, or at least cut it short once it starts coming out in significant quantities.

You may be offered the option of a technique called 'scalp freezing' to try and lessen hair loss. It involves wearing an extremely cold cap for some time before and after a chemotherapy injection. The cold causes the scalp blood vessels to constrict, thereby reducing the drug supply to the hair follicles. It is not suitable for everyone and, although it can work well for some patients, it is not always successful. It does prolong the duration of the chemotherapy session considerably and it can prove uncomfortable for some patients.

● **Other side-effects** Many people feel a little unwell for a day or two after chemotherapy, or sometimes for longer. Tiredness is also common and occasionally it can last for quite a long while after treatment. A rare side-effect of chemotherapy is skin damage at the site of the injection. Some drugs have the ability to cause quite serious ulcers if they leak out of the vein into the surrounding tissues. Nowadays, the staff who administer your chemotherapy are very highly trained and take the utmost care when giving drugs, but this problem can still happen very occasionally. Tell whoever is giving your injection immediately if you experience any pain or discomfort at the injection site while the injection is proceeding, as this may be the first indication of a leak.

Chemotherapy with some drugs can stop the ovaries or testicles working normally. This can result in impaired fertility or infertility, and some women may have an early menopause. Deep-frozen storage of sperms ('sperm banking') is offered to younger men about to receive treatment that may render them infertile.

There are many other potential side-effects of chemotherapy, some being peculiar to particular drugs. However, it is also true to say that most people either do not experience them or do not find them unduly troublesome, or find that they can be satisfactorily treated or even prevented. All side-effects are more likely and more severe in people who are receiving more intensive treatment. They include mouth ulcers, sore eyes, cystitis, diarrhoea, nail changes, numbness of fingers and toes, and rashes. Always report any troublesome symptoms during treatment – quite often there is something that can be done about them. Of course, not all such symptoms are in fact caused by the chemotherapy and other possible causes may need looking into.

Reading about all these possible side-effects can be alarming if you are about to undergo chemotherapy, but it is worth stressing that many people are able to continue with normal life and work for much of the time in between their chemotherapy courses. Indeed, those who do so often seem to cope better with it all. Most people say that chemotherapy was rather less troublesome than they had anticipated.

BONE MARROW TRANSPLANTS

Sometimes chemotherapy is given in very high dosage, with a massive effect on the bone marrow. Such intensive treatment is suitable only for people with some types of cancers, particularly the leukaemias and the lymphomas. It has such a profound effect on the blood that the person being treated needs to be 'rescued' by being given a bone marrow or stem cell transplant. This makes it feasible to give much higher doses of chemotherapy than would otherwise be possible, thereby improving the chance of a cure for people with some cancers.

If you are having a bone marrow transplant using your own marrow, it must be removed before intensive chemotherapy. Alternatively, it may be taken from a 'donor' whose marrow closely matches yours. A close match is important, otherwise it will be 'rejected' later by your immune system. Many donors are close relatives, usually brothers or sisters, but unrelated donors can also sometimes provide marrow that is a good match. The removal or 'harvest' is done by inserting a special needle into the marrow of the bones at the back of the pelvis under general anaesthetic. Only a fairly

RECEIVING NEW MARROW
Healthy bone marrow is injected into the bloodstream via a catheter. The marrow cells then settle in the bone marrow cavities, where they multiply.

small proportion of the total marrow is removed, leaving ample to meet the donor's immediate requirements. It is replaced fairly rapidly by replication of the remaining marrow cells. The removed marrow is frozen and stored until given to you via a drip into a vein after the high-dose chemotherapy. The marrow cells then find their way via the bloodstream to your bones, where they start to manufacture blood cells once again.

STEM CELL TRANSPLANTS

An increasingly common alternative to a bone marrow transplant is what is called a 'stem cell transplant'. This involves removing from your own bloodstream marrow cells (or stem cells) that have been stimulated to leave the marrow by injections of growth factors. A drip is put into a vein in each arm. Blood is taken from one arm into a machine that removes the stem cells and it is then returned via the other drip. The whole procedure takes 3–4 hours. The stem cells are frozen and stored until they are given to you via a drip when required.

HORMONAL TREATMENT

Some cancers depend on hormones for their growth. Hormonal treatments work by preventing cancer cells getting or using the hormones that they need. They tend to have much less effect on normal cells than chemotherapy. However, hormonal treatments are effective only in the treatment of the relatively limited range of cancers that are potentially susceptible to hormonal influences. These are principally those of the breast and prostate, but occasionally cancers of the thyroid and the inner lining of the uterus ('endometrium') will respond to hormonal treatment. Hormonal drugs are often given in tablet form. They work more slowly than chemotherapy and may need to be taken for some months for any effect to become apparent.

TREATING BREAST CANCER HORMONALLY

Tamoxifen, which works by blocking the mechanism by which the hormone oestrogen encourages cancer cells to grow, is by far the most commonly prescribed drug for women with breast cancer. If given as an adjuvant treatment following surgery, it can improve the chance of cure. Adjuvant tamoxifen is usually recommended to be taken for five years. It is mainly effective for those women whose cancer can be shown on laboratory testing to be 'oestrogen-receptor' positive. An oestrogen receptor (also known as 'ER' because of the American spelling 'estrogen') is a complicated chemical molecule found in large amounts on the surface of some cancer cells.

Most women tolerate tamoxifen well, but it can sometimes cause side-effects such as hot flushes, slight weight gain and vaginal discharge. Very infrequently it can cause vaginal bleeding. If you develop this you should tell your doctor so that the reason can be investigated. The cause is usually some benign thickening of the inner lining of the womb but very occasionally there may be a growth that requires treatment.

As well as being used as an adjuvant treatment to increase the chance of cure, tamoxifen can also be used as a palliative treatment. For some women it can relieve symptoms and keep cancers under control for long periods of time. There are a variety of other hormonal drugs that can also be used that have the same aim. They include anastrozole, exemestane, letrozole and megestrol, all given daily in tablet form, and goserelin given by injection beneath the abdominal skin once a month. All palliative hormonal treatments for breast cancer tend to be more effective against slower growing cancers.

In general, these drugs cause few problems, but some women do experience side-effects such as mild nausea, and megestrol can cause weight gain. Although hormonal drugs can keep cancers in remission for long periods in some women, there is a tendency for them eventually to become resistant and escape control. However, if a woman has responded well to one of these drugs, there is quite a good chance that she will respond well to another when the disease relapses.

TREATING PROSTATE CANCER HORMONALLY

This type of cancer is usually highly responsive to hormonal treatments that stop male sex hormones stimulating the cells to divide. At one time this was best achieved by removing the testes, an operation known as 'bilateral orchidectomy'. The same effect can now be achieved, however, by using one of a closely related group of drugs including goserelin and leuprorelin, which in 'slow release' form can be given by injection beneath the abdominal wall skin just once every three months.

These drugs can, however, occasionally stimulate cancer growth in the period immediately after they are first given. This effect can be blocked by taking one of the 'anti-androgen' group of anti-prostate cancer drugs, such as flutamide or cyproterone, in tablet form shortly before the first injection and for about three weeks afterwards.

Hormonal treatments for prostate cancer are usually well tolerated but they can cause loss of sexual desire and impotence. They are quite often recommended for men with more advanced cancers that are not suitable for surgery or radical radiotherapy, but they are also used to shrink down a primary cancer to try to give the surgery or radiotherapy that is to follow a better chance of success.

KEY POINTS

- Drug treatments have the potential to destroy cancer cells wherever they may be.
- There are two main types of drug treatment for cancer: cytotoxic chemotherapy and hormonal treatment.
- It is quite often difficult to predict the response to drug treatments.
- Anyone who is having chemotherapy should report any fever immediately.
- Many people these days find that chemotherapy causes fewer problems than expected.

Further care

Coming to terms with a diagnosis of cancer is not easy for anyone, yet many people do not make sufficient use of all the various kinds of support on offer. It is important that you voice your concerns, whatever they may be, before, during and after treatment. Getting the right kind of supportive care may also make it easier for you to persevere with difficult treatment.

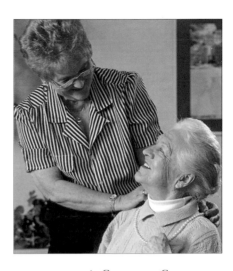

CONTINUING CARE
You may find that you require continued nursing care when you get home. Community or district nurses are available to help with practical tasks, as well as nursing care.

You may need rather more than just treatment directed against your cancer. You may require attention to physical symptoms, which can be very varied. Some will be caused by the cancer, some by treatment and others by something completely unconnected. Often the best way of relieving symptoms is through effective treatment of the underlying cause. If this is not possible, symptoms can usually be abolished or ameliorated in other ways.

You should not feel embarrassed about asking for psychological help. Anxiety and depression are common in people with cancer. Often such feelings are short-lived and not too difficult to cope with, but if they become more troublesome there is usually a variety of different forms of effective help available (see p.90).

Other forms of help that you might possibly need include:
● Professional assistance with rehabilitation
● Help with household tasks and other practical assistance
● Specialised nursing care in hospital, at home or in a hospice
● Financial help: a wide variety of state benefits and charitable financial grants is available for people with cancer and those caring for them at home.

It can quite often take a little while to get over the effects of some of the more intensive treatments with surgery, radiotherapy or drugs. You can usually help your own recovery by eating sensibly and resting whenever you feel tired. Ask your doctor for advice about any plans to return to work or possible changes to your lifestyle. Some people need a fairly long period of convalescence whereas others will be better off returning to normal activity straightaway.

In the longer term, you will probably be advised to lead as normal a life as possible. Obviously, if you have had potentially curative treatment for a smoking-caused cancer, of the larynx or lung for example, you will be strongly advised to give up smoking. Similarly, if you have had treatment for skin cancer you would be wise to avoid excessive exposure to sunlight and use high factor sunscreens. If you try to follow the advice you are given, you will be doing everything in your power to prevent a recurrence of cancer.

For some of those for whom a cure is not possible and who are in need of continuing care, the value of the help that is available from nurses cannot be overstated. Community or district nurses can pay regular visits to patients' homes and they can offer a variety of services including bathing, giving medication and providing support for carers. They may also be able to arrange for the provision of practical aids, for example handrails, or ramps for wheelchairs.

Macmillan nurses have undergone special training in symptom control and counselling. They are often based in hospices but visit patients regularly both in their own homes and in hospital, to offer advice and to check that they are receiving all the care they need. Marie Curie nurses can help out with some of the nursing care at home, thereby providing most valuable relief in some situations, especially at night. Macmillan and Marie Curie nurses offer both advice and practical assistance to family members and other carers. They can usually be contacted via your GP or community nurse.

FOLLOW-UP

Once your treatment is finished, you may well be given 'follow-up' appointments in the hospital outpatient clinic. Usually this is done for very good reasons – to assess the results of treatment, to deal with any side-effects, and to answer questions or give advice on rehabilitation and lifestyle. In some circumstances, however, hospital follow-up, particularly if continued over a long period, is not always the best use of time and energy for either you or your hospital doctor.

One important reason for routine follow-up is the possibility of detecting recurrent cancer at an early and hopefully still curable stage. If your cancer is more advanced and/or incurable, you may be offered routine consultations with the aim of ensuring that your symptoms are being well controlled or that any new ones are treated promptly. Sometimes follow-up can help to ensure proper care for those experiencing side-effects from treatment. But these reasons do not necessarily make it essential to have routine follow-up in hospital. In some circumstances your GP may be happy to share or even supervise follow-up and only send you back to the hospital if there seems to be a problem. This can often work well, and it may spare you unnecessary travel.

However, there are some people for whom follow-up in hospital is essential. This includes particularly those who need specialist internal examinations at regular intervals, for example those who have been treated for 'head and neck', bowel or bladder cancers. You are also likely to need specialist follow-up after curative treatment for certain other cancers, including cervical or testicular cancer, leukaemia, Hodgkin's disease, non-Hodgkin's lymphoma, sarcomas and some skin cancers. Should you have a recurrence of one of these cancers, further treatment may have a greater chance of success if the recurrence is discovered at an early stage. Many women who have had curative treatment for breast cancer need mammograms and thus at least part of their follow-up is conducted in hospital.

Other X-rays and scans are sometimes necessary as part of routine follow-up. Blood tests may also be required, such as blood counts for people who have been treated for leukaemia and 'tumour marker' concentrations for some of those who have had treatment for prostate and testicular cancer.

However, many people do not need any special follow-up tests, although there is, of course, quite a variety of investigations that may be appropriate if there is any cause for concern. Attending for follow-up consultations can understandably be an anxious time for many patients, but nevertheless most patients say that they find regular check-ups reassuring.

FAMILY AND FRIENDS

If you are fortunate enough to have help close at hand from loved ones and close friends, you may well find that they are your main and most valuable source of psychological and practical support.

It is really not surprising that cancer can sometimes put a strain on relationships. This can happen to anyone, but there is a tendency for relationships with previous difficulties to be more vulnerable. Most people find ways to face and overcome new strains and stresses, especially if they are able to share their feelings with each other. For many couples, facing a battle with cancer together makes the relationship even stronger.

Close relatives and friends have an important role to play in helping to maintain your morale, but most people dislike false cheerfulness. If those close to you refuse to consider the possibility of an unfavourable outcome or to recognise your fears and concerns, you may feel less inclined to talk openly to them. Families and friends should not try to 'put on an act' – it is usually best to say and do what comes naturally. Nor should you allow them to turn you into an invalid if you feel that you are perfectly able to live a normal or near-normal life.

You may need more rest than usual, particularly during and for some time after treatment. However, there is usually no reason why you should not continue with your normal activities if you want to and feel up to it. Indeed, many people seem to cope better with treatment and to return more rapidly to normal life afterwards through continuing to be active and involved in the world outside.

Relationships outside the family can also be altered by cancer. Some friends will handle the situation very well and provide valuable understanding, emotional support and practical assistance, whereas others find it difficult to cope. They may become more distant and some even lose touch completely. Most friends will want to help, but some feel uncomfortable and unsure about how best to be of assistance.

The perception that friends are drawing away can be an additional burden, especially if you had expected more of them. It may be helpful to take the initiative by ringing them up or by asking for practical help or for a visit, so that they can be brought back in touch and made to feel useful and needed. Be wary, however, of those who are inclined to make negative comments about your treatment and future prospects based, as they usually are, on relative ignorance.

PSYCHOLOGICAL SUPPORT

Many people do not get this kind of care when they need it, perhaps because they are reluctant to bring up the subject and perhaps because they are not asked about it. It really is worthwhile talking to one of the team responsible for your care if you feel that you are not coping well emotionally with your illness.

Doctors may not always fully appreciate the need of some patients to discuss widely varying aspects of their illness: its treatment, and its impact on their lives and on family and social relationships. Nevertheless, it is an important aspect of their responsibility for you and you should not hesitate to raise matters that concern you, especially if you do not find it easy to talk to family or friends.

EMOTIONAL SUPPORT
Talking over problems and fears with a friend, your GP or a professional counsellor is an essential part of any cancer patient's continuing care.

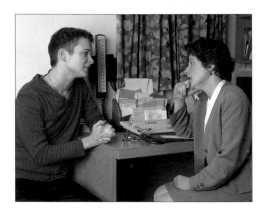

Many people with cancer naturally feel anxious and depressed at times. Many are afraid or feel lonely and isolated. Denial and anger are also common. All these are understandable and can be entirely normal reactions to a disturbing situation. They all tend to be much more marked in the period immediately after being told the diagnosis and around the time of starting treatment. Here 'fear of the unknown' can be an important aspect. As time progresses, these feelings tend to settle.

However, even though later on you may feel that you have come to terms with having an illness that could recur or progress, you can still feel particularly vulnerable every time you have even the slightest symptom, go for a follow-up appointment or hear about someone who has died of cancer. Waiting for the results of tests can also be very stressful. These reactions too tend to diminish with time, but fears can sometimes be still quite profound even years after apparently successful treatment.

Surgery that changes the way you look or the way you see yourself can have a considerable psychological impact. In particular, some people who have had surgical procedures such as mastectomy, laryngectomy or colostomy sometimes feel that they are no longer attractive. They may lose their sex drive and potency. Some do not want to look at themselves naked in the mirror or let their partners see them naked or share a bed with them.

About one in four people with cancer become rather more seriously or persistently depressed. This kind of difficulty is more likely to affect people who are receiving more toxic treatments, younger people, those with more serious cancers, those who have social difficulties and those with a past history of mental problems. Symptoms may include loss of appetite, sleep disturbance, lack of concentration, memory impairment, irritability, feelings of hopelessness and pointlessness of life, panic attacks, sweating, palpitations and shaking. Occasionally patients develop guilt feelings that are often irrational. They may believe, wrongly, that they have brought the disease upon themselves as a result of their lifestyle, or as a result of being of a certain emotional disposition. Others may worry (completely erroneously) that the disease is contagious. Some people feel a stigma and withdraw from social life.

WHERE TO GET HELP

Fortunately, there is much that can be done to help people who are anxious or depressed, or who have other psychological difficulties, so it is important to ask for help when you need it and not try to struggle on alone. What is often most helpful is just being able to talk about your feelings to someone who understands.

People with more serious depression will usually benefit from short-term treatment with an antidepressant drug. Short-term treatment with tranquillisers may help those with severe anxiety. Other types of treatment can also help. For example, some patients benefit from sessions with a therapist who can teach them how to challenge negative thoughts and to use relaxation exercises. Those who have problems with body image following surgery can be helped to see themselves more positively. Specialised psychosexual counselling can be beneficial for people who have lost their sex drive as a result of their illness or treatment. Your doctor can refer you to a clinical psychologist or psychiatrist specialising in this aspect of cancer care if appropriate; if it is not suggested, ask whether this is possible.

Counselling is increasingly becoming part of the care offered in cancer centres. It is important, however, that this is done by suitably experienced medical or paramedical staff, or by dedicated counsellors who have had proper training in counselling, rather than by merely well-motivated volunteers. For this reason, it is better to ask for your doctor's advice rather than finding a counsellor on your own, as the wrong person can sometimes do more harm than good.

Many patients find it extremely helpful to discuss widely ranging aspects of the impact of the disease on their lives, and feel much better for having had this opportunity. Many also benefit from the counselling and spiritual support provided by hospital chaplains or their own priests or ministers.

Emotional as well as practical help is available from various organisations listed in Useful Addresses on p.116. There is also a large number of self-help groups providing support and advice to people with cancer and their families. Many of these groups consist of people who have experienced cancer themselves. You may find it useful to discuss emotional and practical issues with other people who have been through a similar experience to you, although of course no two individuals or families share exactly the same circumstances.

Inevitably, your reaction to your cancer will depend on your personality, which you cannot change. If you have always been an anxious person, you are more likely to dwell on your illness and your fears than someone who is more able to put such concerns aside. However, if you are able to concentrate on getting on with your life and put your cancer behind you as far as possible, you are likely to have a far easier time than if you continue to put your cancer centre stage. It is worthwhile trying to keep a positive attitude and to make each day count.

It is not uncommon for people to say, some years after treatment, that having had cancer led them to re-think their priorities and that, overall, the illness was a positive influence on their lives. The challenge of cancer has enabled some people to become less concerned with trivia and to value more greatly and be grateful for the truly good things in their lives.

PHYSICAL SYMPTOM CONTROL

When you have had cancer, it is easy to attribute any symptom you develop after the diagnosis to cancer, but of course you are still just as susceptible to other complaints – from colds and coughs to rheumatism – as everyone else. Many symptoms have absolutely nothing to do with the cancer or its treatment. However, as a general rule it is sensible to clarify as far as possible the cause of a symptom as this can have a considerable bearing on how it should be best treated.

PAIN CONTROL

It is usually possible to keep pain caused by cancer under control, although sometimes it is necessary to resort to a variety of different measures. Some treatments directed at the cancer itself, such as radiotherapy or drugs, can be very effective in controlling pain. Radiotherapy can be particularly helpful in relieving localised bone pain, usually within a week or two, and very often only a single treatment is required.

As a general rule, pain-killing drugs ('analgesics') need to be taken regularly. Many people are their own worst enemies and wait for the pain to return or to become particularly severe before taking analgesics. It is often much easier to prevent a pain coming on than to make it go away when it is already there. Thus, if you have recurring pain, you should take your analgesic(s) at regular set times, even if you are not actually feeling any pain at that particular time.

There are three broad categories of analgesics: non-opioids, opioids (weak and strong) and additional or 'adjuvant' drugs of various types. Sometimes two types are combined. The correct drug or combination is that which is necessary to control the pain. The non-opioids include paracetamol, aspirin and 'non-steroidal anti-inflammatory drugs' of the type often used for arthritis, such as diclofenac. These anti-inflammatory drugs are often taken in addition to other analgesics and the combination can work very well for some patients.

The weak opioids include co-proxamol and co-codamol. The main strong opioids are morphine given by mouth (orally), diamorphine given by injection and fentanyl given by a skin patch. Tramadol, given either orally or by injection, is an alternative that may be better tolerated by some patients. Oral morphine may be given four-hourly in tablet or liquid form, or 12-hourly using 'slow release' tablets or capsules. If a patient has persistent nausea or vomiting or difficulty with swallowing, it may be helpful to administer diamorphine by slow infusion using a 'syringe driver' (see p.101).

People for whom morphine is prescribed often have reservations about taking it. Sometimes they think that it will stop working if started too soon, or that they will become addicted to it. Neither of these beliefs is correct. Another belief is that the prescription of morphine must indicate that the situation is very serious. This too is a misconception – morphine is simply a very good analgesic that is used when pain is severe. Some people need to take it for many years.

The opioid drugs do have side-effects. Sometimes people become sedated or experience nausea or vomiting when they first start taking them or when the dose is increased, but both these effects tend to wear off fairly rapidly. If necessary, antiemetic drugs can be given. Constipation is a more persisting problem and most people on morphine need to take a softening and stimulant laxative regularly. A dry mouth is also quite common – frequent sips and mouthwashes can help.

Several other measures are available if necessary. These may include taking additional drugs such as steroids, or the antidepressant amitriptyline, which is often helpful in relieving pain caused by pressure on nerves, or nerve damage. For patients with bone pain resulting from metastatic breast cancer or myeloma, bone strengthening 'bisphosphonate' drug treatment may be helpful. It can reduce both the need for pain-relieving radiotherapy and the risk of fracture through areas of weakness.

Referral to a specialist in pain control or in palliative care can be very helpful for some patients. Special pain control techniques are available at pain clinics. Nerve blocks involve the injection of local anaesthetic or other agents near to a nerve to stop it carrying pain impulses to the brain. Transcutaneous electrical nerve stimulation (TENS) machines produce a low electrical current that can be used to stimulate the skin near painful areas and this can also be effective in relieving pain for some patients. No one should accept uncontrolled pain as inevitable.

TENS MACHINE
Transcutaneous electrical nerve stimulation (TENS) is used to relieve pain. The machine is portable, and can be worn while carrying out normal activities.

— CONTROLLING OTHER SYMPTOMS —

Most symptoms can be controlled or at least reduced, sometimes by dealing with the underlying cause, sometimes by treatment directed purely at the symptom and sometimes by a mixture of the two.

LOSS OF APPETITE ('ANOREXIA')

This is a common symptom that may be caused directly by the cancer, treatment with drugs or radiation (particularly when they cause nausea), constipation and psychological upset. Alterations in taste are common in cancer patients and can also play a part in the loss of interest in food.

Many people with anorexia find small, frequent meals more acceptable than larger ones at conventional times, particularly if they are made to look attractive. A glass of sherry before a meal sometimes stimulates appetite, but unfortunately some people also find that they no longer enjoy alcoholic drinks. Drug treatment with progestogens or steroids is sometimes used to stimulate appetite.

BREATHLESSNESS ('DYSPNOEA')

There are a number of possible causes. Some of these involve disruption of the normal functioning of the lungs by the cancer. One of the more common causes is an accumulation of fluid ('pleural effusion') between the outer surface of the lung and the inner surface of the chest wall. The fluid presses on the lung preventing an adequate intake of air. Fortunately, it can be removed very easily and quite comfortably by sucking it out ('aspiration') via a thin needle inserted gently into the fluid through the chest wall. Other causes include primary or secondary growths involving the lung tissue itself, chest infections, anaemia and clots ('pulmonary emboli') in the blood vessels in the lungs. Most can be treated effectively, but if the cause is difficult to deal with, distress can be relieved by morphine, tranquillisers and oxygen.

CONSTIPATION

This is a common problem. It is usually the result of poor dietary intake, analgesics, immobility or combinations of these. Other possible causes include an obstruction in the bowel and a raised blood calcium level. For most patients, prevention is better than cure. Making sure that your diet includes more high-fibre foods such as wholemeal cereals and bread, fresh fruit, pulses and vegetables, and that you keep up your intake of fluids, may be enough to stop you becoming constipated. Some people will need to take laxatives regularly, especially if they are on opioid analgesics. Enemas or suppositories may be necessary to solve the problem in some instances.

EAT MORE FIBRE
Include plenty of fibre-rich foods in your diet such as wholemeal cereals. This will help to prevent constipation.

DIARRHOEA

Unfortunately, diarrhoea is quite often a side-effect of radiotherapy to the abdomen or pelvis, and of some cytotoxic drugs. It usually responds well to a variety of medications, including codeine phosphate and loperamide. However, sometimes it is necessary to stop the anti-cancer treatment for a while to allow the diarrhoea to subside. It is important to make sure that you drink enough fluid to replace what you are losing, and it is usually helpful to cut out or cut down on high-fibre foods and fruit. Patients receiving radiotherapy that would be likely to cause diarrhoea are usually advised to alter their diet preventively.

Normally water is progressively removed from the bowel contents as they move downwards. The contents of the small bowel and the first part of the colon are thus normally rather liquid. This explains why bowel looseness is quite common in people with stomas. Taking methylcellulose can help to firm up the motions. Occasionally diarrhoea can actually be a consequence of constipation, when the more liquid content of the upper bowel seeps past a solid obstruction lower down.

DIFFICULTY WITH SWALLOWING

Difficulty with swallowing ('dysphagia') may be the result of a tumour growing within the oesophagus, or of pressure on the oesophagus from outside, such as by enlarged glands within the centre of the chest. Solids usually cause more problems than liquids with this type of dysphagia. Apart from treatments directed against the cancer itself, rapid relief can often be obtained by inserting a hollow tube or stent down into the oesophagus under sedation or a general anaesthetic ('intubation'). Pain on swallowing can be caused by inflammation resulting from 'heartburn', which is reflux of stomach acid up into the oesophagus, and by chest radiotherapy and infection with thrush ('candidiasis'). Simple and effective remedies are available for all these causes.

LYMPHOEDEMA

Normally tissues are constantly being irrigated by a colourless fluid that flows through small lymphatic channels into lymph nodes, which act as filters and help protect against infection. This fluid, called 'lymph', eventually drains into the bloodstream, but if the lymphatic channels become blocked it can accumulate causing 'lymphoedema' – a boggy swelling of the tissues. It occurs most often in the limbs, and sometimes in the breast.

Lymphatic blockage may be caused by the cancer itself or, a little more commonly, by treatment with surgery or radiotherapy. This is another area where there have been considerable advances in treatment in recent years, including the fitting of appropriate arm or leg stockings and specialised massage.

If you experience this particular problem, you should be able to see one of the many breast care or Macmillan nurses who have been specially trained in lymphoedema care. As tissues affected by lymphoedema tend to be rather vulnerable to infection, you need to try to avoid any injury to the overlying skin and to make sure that you get prompt antibiotic treatment at the first sign of any infection.

NAUSEA AND VOMITING

These symptoms are most commonly caused by drug treatments, particularly analgesics and chemotherapy. Nausea resulting from analgesics such as morphine usually disappears quite quickly even though you continue taking the morphine. Radiotherapy can sometimes cause sickness as well, particularly when given to the abdomen. Nausea and vomiting resulting from chemotherapy or radiotherapy can now quite often be prevented if you are given antiemetic drugs before treatment begins.

Occasionally the cancer itself can give rise to these symptoms, sometimes by causing a rise in the blood calcium concentration ('hypercalcaemia') which can be treated effectively with bisphosphonate drugs. Other causes include constipation, bowel obstruction and metastatic disease in the liver.

If you do develop nausea and vomiting, there is a range of drugs available. They may be given by mouth, by injection, by continuous infusion through a small needle inserted beneath the skin, using a battery powered syringe driver (avoiding the need for repeated injections) or by suppository. Particularly effective are steroids such as dexamethasone and 'HT3-receptor antagonist' drugs such as ondansetron, granisetron and tropisetron. These drugs can have their own side-effects, however. For example, steroids can cause fluid retention, flushing, dyspepsia and insomnia, and HT3-receptor antagonists can cause transient constipation and headache. In many situations less powerful antiemetics such as metoclo-pramide (Maxolon), domperidone (Motilium), haloperidol or cyclizine are sufficient. Quite often certain drugs are used in combination.

Eating little and often may be better than sticking to meal times. It can also be helpful to drink liquids at least an hour before or after meals rather than with the meal.

HOSPICE CARE

Hospices have a tremendous amount to offer when it comes to palliative care. They provide physical symptom relief and psychological and spiritual support, both within the hospices themselves and in people's own homes. Hospice-based care provided by palliative care physicians, specially trained nurses and other health care professionals helps people with cancer to have the best possible quality of life, as well as offering emotional and practical support to family and friends.

If you have never been inside a hospice, you might think they are depressing institutions, but nothing could be further from the truth. They are cheerful places where care is offered in a relaxed and unhurried atmosphere. Most hospice care is given to those who are no longer curable, but many of those who can benefit from it are very far from being terminally ill. Many people enjoy significant improvement in quality of life for prolonged periods as a result of hospice expertise. There is never nothing that can be done.

It is very common for people to be admitted to a hospice for some days for assessment and detailed attention to symptoms, and then to return home much more comfortable. Hospices can also take people in for a few days so as to give their family members or other carers a break. This is sometimes called respite care.

KEY POINTS

- Help is available for many of the physical and psychological problems that affect people with cancer.

- People with cancer often experience symptoms that have nothing to do with the cancer or its treatment.

- Good pain control can be achieved for the great majority of people.

- Pain-killing drugs should usually be taken regularly, not just when the pain begins.

Clinical trials

We have made great progress in cancer care in recent years. There are many reasons for this, including technological developments (such as scanners and improved radiotherapy machines), new anti-cancer drugs and the use of established treatments in different ways, e.g. by giving drugs or radiotherapy in addition to surgery.

Other important factors include the development of drugs that can improve symptom control and reduce the side-effects of some treatments, and a greatly increased understanding of the fundamental nature of the disease.

These developments have resulted in a large number of promising or proven new approaches, many of which are now part of routine care. The speed of change is accelerating: there is an ever-increasing number of new drugs, technologies and concepts arriving on the scene. Unfortunately, however, some new treatments do not live up to their initial promise. What seems to work in the laboratory sometimes has a frustrating tendency not to work in real people. Sometimes a new treatment appears initially to be an improvement, but is found eventually to be no better than what was previously available.

NEW TREATMENTS
The effectiveness and side-effects of a new treatment must be evaluated very carefully before it is used routinely. Patients who take part in clinical trials make an important contribution to medical science.

WHY TRIALS ARE DONE

There is of course only one way to evaluate a new treatment, and that is to try it out on volunteers. It is only because new and experimental treatments were tried out on patients in the past that we are where we are now, but all such research must be conducted and planned meticulously.

A totally new treatment is first evaluated in a fairly small number of patients who are observed very closely indeed, with particular attention being paid to detecting any side-effects. It is at this stage that a drug may be tried at varying dosages, with the aim of discovering the optimum dosage. This is sometimes called a 'phase I' trial.

At a later stage, if the new treatment is showing some possibly useful effect, it may be tried out in a greater number of patients with particular cancers. They are closely monitored to detect both the advantages and disadvantages of treatment in 'phase II' trials.

At a still later stage, the value of a promising new treatment for patients with a particular cancer may be assessed in what is known as a 'randomised controlled', or 'phase III' trial. This trial usually involves comparing the new treatment with what has hitherto been the standard treatment.

In a randomised trial, usually half the patients receive the standard treatment and half the experimental treatment. Who gets what is decided at random, in a process similar to tossing a coin. Sometimes the proportions are slightly different and sometimes more than two treatments are compared, with patients being divided into three or four groups. Everyone involved in a trial gets potentially effective treatment for their illness, but at this stage it will not be clear whether the new treatment is better than the standard approach.

It is important that neither the patient nor the doctor decides which treatment the patient will receive. If there was an element of choice some types of patients might opt for – or be advised to receive – one treatment rather than another. As a result, the two groups might end up being not exactly comparable. Then it might not be possible to tell whether any differences in the response to treatment in the different groups were caused by the particular treatment they had received, or by differences between the patients or by a mixture of the two.

The underlying principle behind a randomised trial is that different treatments are given to groups of patients that are very similar, so that any differences in the way the two groups respond can reasonably be put down to the treatment that they have received.

The similarity between the groups is ensured partly by the random allocation of patients to the different treatments and partly by having large numbers of patients, usually at least hundreds, in the trial. By having large numbers, any differences occurring by chance in the make-up of the patient groups will tend to be ironed out.

As an analogy, it would not be surprising to find a variation in height of several inches within a first form class of secondary school children. However, it would be very surprising if the average height of all first form children in one city was three inches less than in another city not many miles away.

At present, only a fairly small percentage of patients are entered into trials. This is a pity because progress in treatment would come more quickly if more people were included. However, the entering and monitoring of patients in trials are usually fairly time-consuming and often the resources available are not sufficient to cope.

ETHICAL CONSIDERATIONS

A clinical trial can be conducted only with the approval of the local ethical committee, comprising non-medical people and doctors who are not immediately involved in the treatment of the people being entered into the trial. The committee must satisfy itself that there is no evidence that patients will be disadvantaged if entered into the trial.

It is unethical for doctors to invite patients to enter a trial if they already believe that one of the treatments being assessed is superior. Thus, a randomised clinical trial can proceed only if there is genuine uncertainty about which of the treatment options being assessed, if any, is superior. It is quite common for new treatments to be found to be no better than or not as good as already existing treatments, when compared with them in a randomised trial. It is a mistake to assume that all new treatments are better. The progress of trials is kept under close review, and you can be reassured that the trial will be stopped if one treatment is clearly turning out to be better than another.

TAKING PART IN A TRIAL

Patients who take part in a trial may have to attend clinics more often and for longer than if they were not in a trial. This is because very thorough assessments are being made of both treatment efficacy and any side-effects, that would not otherwise be quite so necessary or perhaps even feasible outside a trial.

There is, however, some evidence that, in general, patients treated in trials (whatever treatment they receive) tend to do rather better than those treated outside trials. This may be partly a result of closer monitoring of progress. It may also reflect a tendency for treatment centres and units with particular expertise to be more enthusiastic about entering their patients in trials.

THE CHOICE IS YOURS

If you are invited to join a trial, you are under absolutely no obligation to accept and your refusal will have no effect on the standard of your care: you will still receive the best available conventional treatment. You should not feel that you are under any pressure to join a trial and you must have enough time to make the decision that is right for you. Some people are happy to make their mind up one way or another almost straightaway, but others will want to take away written information about the trial and think about it over a few days.

You can be included in a clinical trial only with your written consent, having received all the information you require about it beforehand, and you are entitled to leave it at any time if you wish.

KEY POINTS

- Progress in the fight against cancer depends on patients being treated in clinical trials.
- All clinical trials are very carefully vetted.
- Patients in a trial cannot receive any treatment that is known to be inferior.
- Patients in trials tend to do better, whatever treatment they receive.
- A patient can be entered into a trial only with his or her informed consent.

Complementary treatments

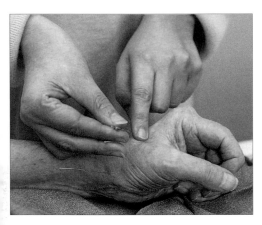

In recent years, increasing numbers of people with cancer have chosen to try 'complementary' treatments in addition to what may be called orthodox or 'mainstream' medical care. Many of these people say that they have benefited from complementary medicine as far as their emotions and general sense of well-being are concerned.

CHINESE MEDICINE
Although we do not fully understand how acupuncture really works, some cancer patients find that it helps to alleviate pain.

COMPLEMENTARY THERAPIES

Many different treatments may be offered under the complementary medicine umbrella, and most have been developed outside mainstream medicine. You will normally have to pay for them although some, such as aromatherapy massage, are now being offered free in some hospitals and hospices.

ACUPUNCTURE

An ancient form of Chinese medicine in which fine needles are inserted at specific points. A wide variety of techniques is available, ranging from a traditional Chinese approach to Western adaptations. There is evidence that acupuncture may help in pain control although this has not been scientifically proven.

HOMOEOPATHY

Based on the principle that 'like cures like', homoeopathic remedies contain infinitesimal quantities of substances that, it is believed, would in larger amounts produce similar symptoms to the illness being treated. Practitioners believe that these help the body to heal itself. However, there is no scientific evidence of benefit from homoeopathy as an anti-cancer treatment.

MASSAGE

Gentle massage can help patients to relax and may help relieve muscular pain and stiffness, leading to a feeling of improved well-being. Aromatherapy involves aromatic essential oils being massaged gently into the skin. Reflexology is another type of massage, given to the feet. Massage directly over a cancer that can be felt near the surface is probably best avoided.

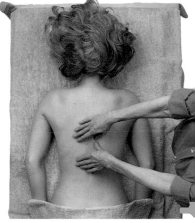

MEDITATION

This involves calm contemplation, controlling or directing your thoughts and emotions by using one of a range of techniques to shut out distraction. It can help some individuals achieve a sense of inner peace and relief of anxiety, and possibly some relief of pain.

A RELAXING EXPERIENCE
A massage is a pleasurable experience, and can help to promote a patient's well-being by inducing calm and reducing stiffness and pain.

RELAXATION

A number of techniques is available, all designed to encourage a sense of physical and mental calm, and to combat anxiety and tension.

SPIRITUAL HEALING

Healers may have differing spiritual or religious beliefs, but all claim to transfer some form of healing energy. Healing is usually considered to come from a divine origin, through prayer and meditation. Healing may or may not involve touch and some healers actually work from a distance. Those receiving healing may experience relaxation and a feeling of inner peace.

VISUALISATION

This involves using the imagination to conjure up images that the individual may find helpful as an aid to relaxation, meditation or symptom control. Some people find it helpful to imagine their immune system fighting their cancer.

DIETS AND VITAMINS

It makes good sense to try to maintain a 'normal' or 'healthy' balanced diet, sufficient in protein, calories, vitamins and fibre. A great number of different special diets have been advocated over the years. Large amounts of vitamins have been quite a common feature. However, although special diets may sound a good idea, there is little evidence that they can influence the chance of cure or help keep a cancer under control.

Some people feel that by going on special diets they are being constructively involved in the fight against their cancer and that this helps them psychologically. Unfortunately, others find their diet unpleasant and it impairs their quality of life.

VITAMIN SUPPLEMENTS

Carrots often feature prominently in special diets. They are rich in beta-carotene, which is converted to vitamin A in the digestive tract. There is some evidence suggesting that low dietary levels of vitamin A or beta-carotene may lead to an increased risk of cancer, and there are studies in progress looking at whether supplements of beta-carotene or related substances known as retinoids can reduce cancer incidence.

Retinoids have been shown to have some efficacy in the treatment of some human tumours but, like high doses of natural vitamin A, they can cause side-effects, including nausea, vomiting, headache, skin changes and psychiatric disturbance. There is no good evidence that they can improve the chance of cure. Consuming large amounts of carotene-containing foods can occasionally cause the skin to turn yellow.

It has been suggested that vitamin C can render normal tissues less susceptible to destruction by chemicals released by cancer cells. It was reported in one study that patients given high doses of vitamin C lived longer than expected, but subsequent randomised trials have provided no evidence of benefit.

HERBAL MEDICINE

It should not be forgotten that various anti-cancer drugs of proven efficacy used in mainstream medicine originate from plants. Herbal medicines have considerable appeal to some, stemming particularly from their being thought of as 'natural'. Outside orthodox oncology, several herbal preparations have been claimed to have particular benefit for cancer patients. One example is iscador, a fermented mistletoe extract given by injection. It is claimed that it exerts its beneficial effects both by killing cancer cells and by altering beneficially the body's immune system. Although there have been anecdotal claims of efficacy, there is no evidence to support this from properly conducted clinical trials. Another example is laetrile. The principal ingredient of this substance is amygdalin, found in apricot stones and almonds. It has been suggested that laetrile causes toxic hydrogen cyanide to be released selectively within cancer cells. There is no scientific justification for this hypothesis and unfortunately careful clinical study has again produced no evidence of efficacy.

THE IMPORTANCE OF THE MIND

There is quite a common belief among complementary therapists that a person's psychological make-up is relevant to the development and subsequent course of their cancer.

MIND POWER
There is much controversy over whether the mind can play a significant part in determining the outcome of a serious disease such as cancer.

It has been suggested that some people are cancer prone by virtue of their personality, but there is no good scientific evidence to support this. Nor is there conclusive evidence that the psyche influences survival chances for cancer patients. There is some evidence that it can, and quite a few mainstream oncologists believe that it does, but even if psychological factors do exert some influence on outcome, this is not necessarily of any help in practice.

Some complementary therapists believe that psychological stress can encourage the development of cancer, and that it is possible to enable people with the disease to fight it effectively by changing their frame of mind. The role of stress as a causative agent remains a controversial issue, with different studies arriving at different conclusions, but so far the evidence to support the theory that psychological treatment offers any benefits in fighting the cancer, over and above that of improving psychological well-being, is inconclusive.

There have been numerous reports on the part played by a person's innate psychological characteristics, sometimes suggesting that those who are able freely to express emotion or distress tend to survive longer than those who suppress or deny their emotional feelings. One study of women with breast cancer who underwent psychological assessment at the diagnosis of their illness found that those who had reacted to cancer by denial or who had a 'fighting spirit' did rather better than those who had responded with stoic acceptance or feelings of hopelessness. However, another study failed to show a relationship between such psychological factors and outcome. Nor did social factors such as friendships, marital history or job satisfaction have any influence.

A study on a small number of women with advanced breast cancer demonstrated increased survival in those randomised to participate in weekly supportive group therapy and self-hypnosis for pain control. Another small study demonstrated increased survival in people with melanoma skin cancer who had received 'psycho-educational intervention' including stress management, enhancement of coping skills and supportive group psychotherapy. Such results are very interesting, but other studies have failed to show that this type of treatment makes people live longer. More research needs to be done before we have conclusive results, one way or the other.

CONSIDERING TREATMENT

There are more things in heaven and earth than are currently dreamed of by practitioners of mainstream medicine. However, it should not be forgotten that most of the progress that has been made in the fight against cancer has been as a result of critical scientific evaluation.

Most complementary treatments have not been exposed to or have not withstood the rigours of scientific testing. Nevertheless, there is no doubt that many people say that they feel better as a result of complementary therapy. Although the extent to which this is the result of the treatment itself remains controversial, it seems likely that there are other less tangible factors at work. A complementary therapist is often willing and able to give you as much time and personal attention as you want – something that is not always possible for your doctors. It is also true that many people simply feel better for trying to do something to help themselves, especially when conventional medicine may have little to offer them.

Whether or not complementary treatments can influence the outcome as far as the cancer is concerned is obviously a very important issue. Many of those offering and receiving them believe that the chance of survival will be improved, but there is little evidence to support this. There is understandable concern about people with cancer having their hopes raised unrealistically.

Complementary treatments are often considered as part of a 'holistic' or 'whole person' approach to care, implying that conventional medicine is more concerned with the disease than with the patient. The pressures on the service and the resulting constraints on time may quite often result in patients getting this impression, but most doctors would maintain that good conventional medicine has always been holistic.

Most complementary treatments for people with cancer in Britain are offered entirely in good faith. However, you also need to be aware of the possibility of being exploited commercially by the unscrupulous. Marketing strategies for non-orthodox treatments include both giving complex pseudo-scientific rationales and making superficially attractive conceptual claims, neither of which stand up to close inspection. Non-conventional methods may be hailed as 'natural', and much may be made of the toxicity of some conventional treatments, but some alternative treatments can themselves be toxic or unpleasant.

If you are thinking about some kind of complementary therapy, it is worth mentioning this to your doctor; who may be able to give you some useful advice. In any case, your doctor should know about any treatment you are having in order to take it into account when assessing your progress, or possibly when faced with new symptoms or other changes in your condition.

You should be wary of any therapist who says or implies that their treatment can cure you or shrink the cancer, and you should make sure that you are clear in your own mind about what you expect the treatment to do for you. Do not stop taking any conventional treatment without first discussing it with your doctor.

KEY POINTS

- People often feel better psychologically after having complementary therapy.

- Complementary therapies have not yet been proved to be of benefit in improving survival or the chance of cure.

- Most complementary medicine is offered in good faith, but you should be wary of being exploited by unscrupulous practitioners while you are at your most vulnerable.

Useful Addresses

England
Cancer Bacup
3 Bath Place
Rivington Street
London EC2A 3JR
Cancer Support Service:
Tel: (0207) 613 2121
(information)
(0207) 696 9003 (booklets
about different types of cancer
and treatments)
Freephone: (0808) 800 123
Website:
www.cancerbacup.org.uk
Provides advice and
information about all aspects
of cancer as well as emotional
support for cancer patients
and their families.

Bristol Cancer Help Centre
Grove House
Cornwallis Grove
Clifton
Bristol BS8 4PG
Tel: (0117) 9809505
Pioneering centre offering
complementary help for
physical, psychological and
spiritual problems. People with
cancer are offered relaxation,
healing, visualisation,
counselling, diets, meditation,
music and art therapy.
Charges are made for services,
but discretionary financial
assistance is available.

Cancer and Leukaemia in Childhood (CLIC)
12–13 King Square
Bristol BS2 8JH
Tel: (0117) 924 8844
Offers support to children
with cancer and their families,
including financial help and
'home from home'
accommodation. Provides
domiciliary care nurses to
help with care at home.

Cancer Care Society
11 The Cornmarket
Romsey
Hampshire SO51 8GB
Tel: (0117) 942 7419
An organisation of people with
cancer, relatives and friends
who offer help and support.
Trained counsellors also
provide telephone and personal
counselling. A telephone link
service allows people to talk to
others in similar situations.

Cancerlink
11–21 Northdown Street
London N1 9BN
Freephone: (0808) 8080000
Freephone (Asian language
line): (0800) 590415;
Freephone (Mac helpline for
young people): (0800) 591028
Provides information and
emotional support for people
with cancer and their families.

Consumers' Advisory Group for Clinical Trials
Acacia House
17 Devonshire Avenue
Grimsby
Lincolnshire DN32 0BW
Tel: (01472) 752045
Aims to improve public
understanding of clinical trials.
It also brings together
members of the lay public and
doctors to improve the design
of trials.

Crossroads Caring for Carers
10 Regent Place
Rugby
Warwickshire CV21 2PN
Tel: (01788) 573653
Provides respite care.
Attendants come into the
home to give the carer a break.

CRUSE – Bereavement Care
Cruse House
126 Sheen Road
Richmond
Surrey TW9 1UR
Tel: (0208) 940 4818
Offers help via local branches
to bereaved people. Individual
and group counselling are
provided and also practical
advice. A wide variety of
publications and leaflets are
available.

The Hospice Information Service
St Christopher's Hospice
51–59 Lawrie Park Road
Sydenham SE26 6DZ
Tel: (0208) 778 9252
Provides information on hospice services in Britain and throughout the world. Publishes a directory of services giving details of hospices, home care teams and hospital support teams.

Institute for Complementary Medicine
PO Box 194
London SE16 7QZ
Tel: (0207) 237 5165
Provides names of practitioners of various kinds of complementary medicine.

Macmillan Cancer Relief
15–19 Britten Street
London SW3 3TZ
Tel: (0207) 351 7811
A national charity dedicated to improving the quality of life for people with cancer, and their families. It funds Macmillan Nursing Services, for home care, hospital and hospice support. Offers financial help.

Marie Curie Cancer Care
28 Belgrave Square
London SW1X 8QG
Tel: (0207) 235 3325
Runs Marie Curie nursing homes and provides a community nursing service day and night. Involved also in research and the education of

health professionals in cancer care and prevention.

National Cancer Alliance
PO Box 579
Oxford OX4 1LB
Tel: (01865) 793566
An organisation of cancer patients, their relatives and friends, and health care professionals, working together to improve cancer services, treatment and care throughout the United Kingdom. Provides information about good care and services and produces a Directory of Cancer Specialists.

Sargent Cancer Care for Children
Griffin House
161 Hammersmith Road
London W6 8SG
Tel: (0208) 752 2800
Supports young people under the age of 21 with cancer and their families, through counselling, practical care and financial help. There are also holiday homes in Scotland and Northern Ireland where families can enjoy a break.

Scotland
Tak Tent Cancer Support
Flat 5, 30 Shelley Court
Gartnavel Complex
Glasgow G12 OYN
Tel: (0141) 2111930
Provides information, emotional support and counselling. There are support groups throughout Scotland.

Wales
Tenovus Cancer Information Centre
PO Box 88
College Buildings
Courtenay Road
Splott
Cardiff CF24 2ZA
Freephone: (0800) 526527
Provides information, emotional support and counselling. Counselling is available in both Welsh and English languages.

Ireland
The Irish Cancer Society
5 Northumberland Road
Dublin 4
Tel: 1 668 1855
Provides information on all aspects of cancer, home care, rehabilitation programmes and support groups.

Ulster Cancer Foundation
40–42 Eglantine Avenue
Belfast BT9 6DX
Freephone: (0800) 7833339
Provides information, counselling, rehabilitation and other support services.

Index

Acknowledgements

PUBLISHER'S ACKNOWLEDGEMENTS

Dorling Kindersley would like to thank the following for their help and participation in this project:

Production Controller Michelle Thomas; **DTP** Jason Little; **Consultancy** Dr. Sue Davidson; **Indexing** Indexing Specialists, Hove; **Administration** Christopher Gordon.

Photography: Paul Mattock (p.98); Ian Parsons.(p.49, p.103); Department of Medical Illustration, Royal United Hospital, Bath (p70)

Picture Research Andy Samson; **Picture Librarian** Charlotte Oster.

PICTURE CREDITS

The publisher would like to thank the following for their kind permission to reproduce their photographs. Every effort has been made to trace the copyright holders. Dorling Kindersley apologises for any unintentional omissions and would be pleased, in any such cases, to add an acknowledgement in future editions.

Dr Gordon, Anatomic Pathology Division of Department of Pathology and Laboratory Medicine, University of Pennsylvania Medical Center p 30r; **Sally and Richard Greenhill** p.108; **Robert Harding Picture Library** p.52, p.85 (Dick Dickinson/Int'l Stock); **Science Photo Library** p.24; p 78 (Simon Fraser/Royal Victoria Infirmary, Newcastle; p.22 (King's College School of Medicine), p.3, p.9 (Mehau Kulyk); p.38bla, p.38bl (Dr. P. Marazzi); p.90 (Claire Paxton and Jacqui Farrow); p.19 (Chris Priest); p.33 (Department of Clinical Radiology, Salisbury District Hospital); p11tl (L.Willatt, East Anglian Regional Genetics Service); **The Stock Market** p.60; **Telegraph Colour Library** p.7 (H. Sykes).